Glow Through the Change

A Holistic Guide to Gua Sha: Empowering You to Navigate Menopausal Symptoms With Confidence

Divya Jagtiani

Glow Through the Change
A Holistic Guide to Gua Sha: Empowering You to Navigate Menopausal Symptoms With Confidence
© 2025 SHANTI 3 LIMITED

All rights reserved.

No part of this book may be reproduced, stored in a retrieval system or transmitted in any form or by any means (electronic, mechanical, photocopy, recording, scanning or other) except for brief quotations in critical reviews or articles, without the prior written permission of the publisher.

ISBN: 9781068276903 Paperback

Published by: Inspired By Publishing

Disclaimer

This book is intended for general informational and educational purposes only. It does not constitute medical, nutritional, or professional advice, and should not be relied upon as such.

The author is not a licensed medical practitioner or nutritionist. Readers should consult a suitably qualified professional for individually tailored advice regarding any health, wellbeing, or lifestyle changes. The content of this book offers general guidance and may not be applicable to individual circumstances.

This book is not intended for individuals with specific medical conditions or diagnoses. Anyone with a known or suspected health issue should seek advice from an appropriate medical professional before acting on any information contained herein.

The author and publisher expressly disclaim all liability for any loss, injury, or harm resulting from the use or misuse of the information contained in this book. By reading and using this book, you agree to take full responsibility for your actions and waive any claims against the author or publisher.

Any success stories or outcomes shared in this book are anecdotal and may not be typical. Some may be fictionalised or dramatised for illustrative purposes. Individual results will vary, and no guarantees of outcomes are expressed or implied.

A full bibliography is provided for reference.

Certain aspects of this book were assisted by artificial intelligence tools, including but not limited to language refinement and image development. All final content, creative direction and responsibility remain with the author.

The author reserves the right to revise or update the content at any time and makes no representations or warranties regarding its accuracy, completeness, or relevance, and accepts no responsibility or liability whatsoever for any loss or consequence arising from its use.

DEDICATION

To my Nana

Who always said,

"Count your Blessings,

Think Positive,

Always be Happy," and

"Divya, you can do anything."

Nana, this book is for you.

Calling all Goddesses: It's time to claim your power.

CONTENTS

INTRODUCTION   1

Part 1 All About Menopause,
         The Symptoms And Your Skin

Chapter 1   DIVINE FEMININE ENERGY   15

Chapter 2   MENOPAUSAL SKIN   39

Chapter 3   LET'S TALK ABOUT
            HOT FLUSHES   61

Part 2 All About Gua Sha

Chapter 4   AWAKEN YOUR INNER GODDESS
            WITH GUA SHA   93

Chapter 5   GUA SHA TECHNIQUES   109

Chapter 6   RELIEF FROM COMMON
            MENOPAUSAL SYMPTOMS   135

| Chapter 7 | ENHANCING GUA SHA WITH THE RIGHT FACIAL OIL **157** |

Part 3 **The Glow-Up Plan**

| Chapter 8 | THE ESSENTIAL ROLE OF NUTRITION IN NAVIGATING MENOPAUSE **183** |

| Chapter 9 | DESIGNING YOUR ROUTINE **209** |

| Chapter 10 | EMBRACE YOUR GLOW WITH YOUR MENOPAUSE IKIGAI AND DOPAMINE MENU **229** |

CONCLUSION Embracing Your Glow **249**

BIBLIOGRAPHY **255**

REFERENCES **259**

APPENDIX 1 Your Guide To Menopausal Skincare: Be Confident, Informed and In Control **263**

APPENDIX 2 50 Essential Ingredients for Menopause-Friendly Meals: Your Ultimate Cheat Sheet **270**

INTRODUCTION

Menopause is often spoken about in whispers, if at all. For too long, it has been treated as something to dread, something to hide, something a woman must endure in silence. But not here. Not in this space.

This is where we rewrite the narrative. This is where you rise. Here, you are not alone, and you are not invisible.

My journey into the world of menopause began not with a textbook, but with a moment. One that was raw, uncomfortable and unforgettable.

How do I even bring this up? I thought, nervously fidgeting with my fingers as Mum rambled on about her plans for the day.

I could barely concentrate over the heavy, pungent smell filling my bedroom. It smelled terrible. I cringed, knowing the words had to come out somehow. But how do you tell your own mother that she smells awful without crushing her?

With a deep breath, I interrupted her mid-sentence, heart pounding. "Mum, I don't know how to say this…" I said, slowly. "No offence, but there's a really strong smell coming from you…"

Mum paused, blinking at me with confusion. "What do you mean?" she asked, her voice a mix of surprise and defensiveness. My stomach tightened as I shifted uncomfortably.

"Your sweat… it stinks," I said quietly, feeling the heat rise in my cheeks. The words hung in the air, heavy and awkward. For a moment, everything was silent, as if the world had stopped to listen in on the worst conversation of my life.

Then it happened. Her face crumpled and tears welled up in her eyes. She looked at me like I'd just kicked her. "I've had three showers today!" she sobbed, her voice cracking. "I feel so hot all the time! I don't know what to do with these hot flushes!"

My heart sank. Of course. The menopause. I'd heard her mention it in passing, but never really thought much about what she was going through. Now I felt like the worst person alive.

"Mum, I'm so sorry, I didn't mean to upset you," I rushed to say, grabbing her hand. "I didn't realise. I just… I didn't know."

She wiped her eyes with the back of her hand, still sniffling. "I've been trying everything. It's like no matter what I do, I can't stop sweating," she said, her voice fragile. "It's humiliating."

I squeezed her hand, guilt gnawing at me. "I didn't mean to hurt your feelings. I just wanted to let you know. Maybe we can figure something out together? There's got to be something that can help."

Mum nodded, looking at me through watery eyes. "I just feel so embarrassed. It's like I'm losing control of my own body."

"You're not alone, Mum," I said gently. "We'll figure it out. Together."

Her tear-streaked face softened slightly, and for the first time since this disastrous conversation began, I felt a glimmer of relief. Maybe, just maybe, I could find a way to help her after all.

And that was the moment everything changed.

That conversation set me on a path I never expected, one that led me deep into the world of menopause. As a lawyer, research was second nature to me. I threw myself into medical journals, studies and holistic health practices. But as a daughter, it was different. This wasn't just research; it was personal. I wasn't just reading about symptoms, I was witnessing them. I wasn't just looking at solutions, I was searching for ways to ease my mother's suffering.

My name is Divya, a former structured finance lawyer, certified Theta Healer, gua sha enthusiast and the founder of SHANTI[3], a skincare and wellness brand rooted in the Sanskrit philosophy of peace of body, mind and spirit. I help women, especially those going through menopause, feel empowered, confident in their skin and supported in both physical and emotional healing. I guide those who are ready to reclaim their skin, their energy and their self-worth, helping them glow with confidence from the inside out.

But why write a book on menopause if I'm not going through it myself?

Yes, ageing is inevitable, but I believe in taking control of my body and mind rather than waiting for menopausal symptoms to appear. I wrote this book first for my mother, then for my future self and finally, for *you*. Because no woman should have to go through this transition feeling lost, unsupported or invisible. This journey is shared, and this book invites you to feel seen, heard and held. This book is here to guide you whether you're just starting to notice changes, experiencing menopause first-hand or preparing for what's ahead.

Throughout this book, you'll discover simple, supportive tools to reconnect with your body, nourish your spirit and reclaim your glow. From skincare rituals and mindset shifts to nutrition tips and sleep strategies, you'll learn to honour this stage of life as a sacred transformation instead of viewing it as a slow decline.

The Awakening of Your Divine Feminine

Close your eyes for a moment and ask yourself:

Am I a Goddess?

If your answer is "yes," how beautiful. You already glow with the light of knowing who you are. You walk through life radiant in your energy, your presence, your truth. You may not need this book, but I hope it reminds you just how powerful you truly are.

And if your answer is "no," then I invite you to lean in.

Would you like to feel what it's like to move through the world with magnetic grace? To wake up each day grounded in purpose, glowing from the inside out? To hold the undeniable power of your divine feminine energy, not as a fantasy, but as your daily truth?

A woman rooted in her feminine power moves with intention and speaks with conviction. She knows her worth and does not seek permission to shine. She is not rattled by ageing, nor dimmed by the whispers of societal expectation. She is anchored in her own rhythm, radiant in her own skin.

She doesn't just enter a room; she shifts the energy in it. Her sparkle can't be manufactured. It's that indescribable *je ne sais quoi*, an energy that draws others in without her saying a word. Women admire her. Men are magnetised by her. But most importantly, she sees herself clearly. That is her superpower.

Maybe you've lost your sparkle, or maybe you've never fully felt it before.

But I promise you, it's there.

When I think of this kind of energy in its purest form, I think of Marilyn Monroe. Not the Hollywood glamour, but the woman who knew how to turn her light on like a switch. She could walk through the streets of New York unnoticed, simply dressed, hidden in plain sight.

And then, something would shift.

Her story may seem unexpected, but it holds a profound truth about embodied feminine power.

As the story goes, she once turned to her friend Amy Greene as they walked outside and, with a playful glint in her eye, asked, "Do you want to see me become her?" Amy nodded. In that instant, Marilyn changed. She didn't alter her clothes or raise her voice. She simply *became*. With a tilt of her chin and an inner shift, the city stopped. Cars slowed. Heads turned. A moment ago, she was just a woman on the sidewalk. Now, she was *Marilyn Monroe*. Her transformation wasn't about performance; it was about presence.

That is goddess energy. The ability to command a moment not through effort, but through embodiment.

And here's what I want you to know: You have that same switch within you.

If menopause has felt like it's dimmed your light, made you question your power or left you feeling unseen, please know you are not alone.

And more than that, know this: You have not lost your glow. This is your time to remember what has always lived within you.

In 2025, approximately 1.1 billion women will be going through menopause worldwide.[1] That's 13.4% of the global population. Every woman will spend around 30% of her life in menopause. So why is it still treated like a taboo? Why do so many women suffer in silence, left to figure it out on their own?

If you're frustrated by how you're feeling...
If your family doesn't understand what you're going through...
If your symptoms look different from your friends' and you don't know why...
If you're exhausted from juggling responsibilities while trying to make sense of it all...
If you're scared of getting older, of losing yourself in the process...

If any of the above resonates with you, I'm here to tell you: You are not meant to just get on with it. You can tap into your goddess energy and glow through the change. Every woman carries it, but many won't awaken it. This is your time to reclaim your fire.

You're going to elevate your mindset to that of a woman fully in her power. Some may be afraid of becoming unrecognisable, of shedding old identities. But that is where your evolution begins.

Women who embrace their feminine power are unfazed by menopause. They know they are thriving every day, in every stage, in every season. They are the prize.

As such, a woman in her power knows menopause is not something to endure, but rather, something to embrace. It's a new chapter, one where you get to redefine what ageing looks and feels like on your terms.

This book is not for you if you're looking for a dense, medical textbook filled with jargon or a one-size-fits-all quick fix. It's not for those who aren't open to making small but meaningful changes or who see menopause as something to simply suffer through rather than a transition they can take charge of. But if you're ready to step into your light, to embrace your evolution and to glow, then this is exactly the book you need.

We're here to flip the narrative on menopause, from something difficult and uncomfortable to a powerful opportunity for renewal, growth and self-discovery. In Traditional Chinese Medicine, menopause is known as the "second spring", a time of rebirth where you step into a new phase of life with wisdom, confidence and empowerment. This isn't an ending; it's a fresh beginning, a chance to embrace change on your own terms and redefine what this stage of life means to you.

This book is for you if you want to feel confident and empowered, if you want to reconnect with your divine feminine energy as you glow through the change.

This book is your guide to thriving, not just surviving. You'll learn how to:

- Support your skin through menopause with gua sha techniques (my personal favourite)

- Soothe hot flushes naturally and design a routine that works for you

- Optimise your nutrition with the Essential Ingredients for Menopause-Friendly Meals

- Build small but powerful habits to feel energised, clear-minded and in control

- Shift your mindset from pain to power

Throughout each chapter, you'll find gentle rituals, practical tools and holistic insights to bring your power back home.

If you're looking for practical, no-nonsense advice to help with hot flushes, bloating and menopausal skin changes, without feeling overwhelmed, then you're in the right place. This book is for you if you want to feel good in your skin, both inside and out, with simple lifestyle shifts, self-care rituals and beauty tips that empower you to radiate confidence. It's for those who see menopause not as an ending but as an opportunity to reset, renew and step into a new phase of life feeling empowered.

Would you like to take control of your menopause journey and feel empowered every step of the way? Would you like to tap into your inner radiance?

Become your own doctor with the Menopause Symptoms Tracker. It will help you identify patterns in your symptoms and understand what your body truly needs.

Become your own nutritionist, selecting foods with intention to nourish your body, mind and soul.

Become your own gua sha masseuse, using this powerful technique to soothe menopausal skin, ease hot flushes, support digestion, reduce bloating and create a daily ritual of self-care and relaxation.

Become your own master goal-setter, using the 12-week calendar to transform your routine, fuel motivation and step into each day with purpose.

Become your own sleep specialist, designing an evening ritual that supports deep, high-quality sleep so you wake up refreshed and energised.

You already have everything within you to navigate this transition with confidence, strength and grace. Now it's time to claim it.

You can embody your goddess energy at any stage of your life. Women who embrace this energy understand their bodies.

They know how to manage their menopausal symptoms effectively. They prioritise self-care, nourish their bodies, minds and spirits with healthy habits, movement and rest. They embrace emotional wellbeing. They don't just manage anxiety; they transmute it into confidence. They are compassionate and supportive. They feel empowered every single day.

They don't see menopause as a struggle. They see it as a sacred return, a powerful chapter filled with strength, wisdom and self-discovery.

Instead of just going through the change, you're glowing through it. Let this be your moment. Let this be your rise.

Calling all Goddesses: Step into your light, take control of your journey and glow through the change.

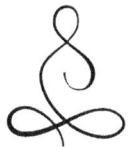

Part 1

ALL ABOUT MENOPAUSE, THE SYMPTOMS AND YOUR SKIN

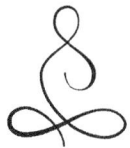

Chapter 1
DIVINE FEMININE ENERGY

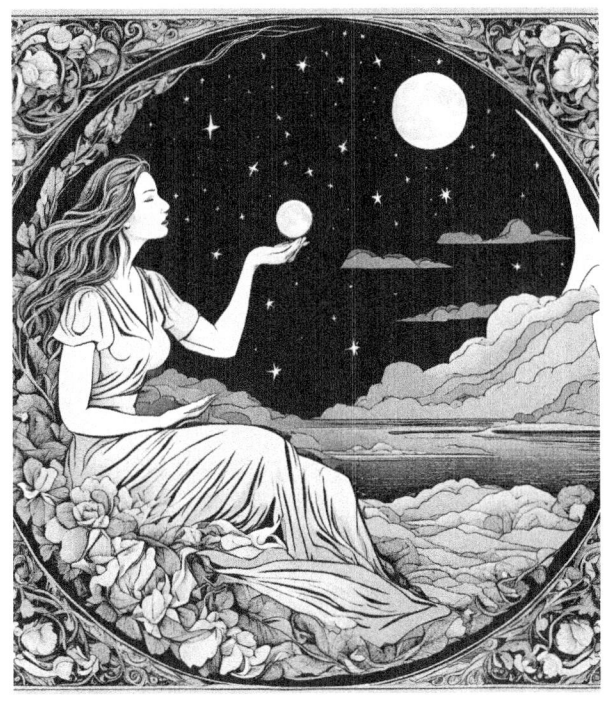

Before we dive into the practical tools and teachings, let's begin where all true transformation starts – within. Menopause may be a biological transition, but how you experience it is deeply shaped by how you see yourself.

This chapter invites you to reconnect with the truth that's been inside you all along: your divine feminine power.

Goddess Energy

Have you ever wondered why some women just seem radiant, confident and stand strong in their feminine power? Divine feminine energy isn't just about how you look or what you do. It's about how you think. It's a mindset, a way of carrying yourself, a deep-rooted belief that you are worthy and powerful.

You don't wait to feel like her. You decide to become her, and then you show up, as her, every single day.

Tapping into your divine feminine power is about unlocking the illuminated, powerful and magnetic force that already exists within you. It's not about becoming someone new, but about fully embracing the woman you already are. It's the quiet confidence that commands a room without saying a word, the effortless grace that moves through life's challenges with resilience and the deep self-assurance that allows you to stand tall, unapologetically owning your worth. This energy is what makes you feel alive in your own skin, connected to your desires and in tune with your intuition.

It's the glow that comes not from external validation but from the fire that burns within, a fire that never truly goes out, no matter what stage of life you're in.

Like Norma Jeane becoming Marilyn Monroe as she walks the streets of New York, you can activate this energy at any time. The world reflects the energy you embody. When you choose to own your presence, walk with confidence, and think like a goddess, the world responds. That is feminine magnetism – the ability to transform your reality in a matter of seconds, not by changing who you are, but by stepping into your power.

Think Like a Goddess, Become the Goddess

How do you do this?

By shifting the way you speak to yourself. By questioning the old narratives that no longer serve you. By recognising that the only opinion that truly matters is your own.

For too long, you have carried thoughts that were never truly yours, beliefs imposed by society, expectations shaped by others, and doubts planted in your mind. But you are not your thoughts. A woman rooted in her power knows this, and she chooses which thoughts to keep and which to release.

So when a thought like *"I am afraid I am no longer beautiful as I grow older"* appears, she does not accept it as truth. Instead, she pauses. She questions it:

Is this really true?

Is this belief my own, or something I was taught to believe?

Does holding onto this thought serve me?

And then, she rewrites the story.

Instead of clinging to a thought that lowers her energy, she replaces it with one that elevates her spirit:

"I love myself. I am worthy. I am enough simply because I exist."

A woman in her divine energy knows that her mind is a garden, and her thoughts are the seeds. She has the power to cultivate beauty or allow weeds to take over. Whenever a negative thought appears, she gently removes it, making space for positivity, wisdom and confidence to bloom.

The energy you carry is the energy you attract. When you begin to embody the power, grace and confidence of your feminine self, everything around you shifts to meet you at that level. You stop seeking permission to shine and start trusting your power. You set boundaries with ease, walk with purpose and carry a presence that is both strong and soft. Beauty is not just in how you look but in how you move, how you speak and the energy you bring into a room.

It's about feeling sensual, vibrant and alive for no one but yourself. It's about allowing joy, pleasure and fulfilment into your daily life, whether through how you move, how you dress or how you honour yourself. You don't have to chase anything.

Because *you* are the magic.

How This Mindset Will Guide You Through Menopause

This divine feminine mindset is the foundation upon which the rest of this journey will unfold. As we move through the chapters ahead, you'll see how this transformation isn't just about changing how you think. Rather, it's about changing how you experience menopause. Menopause is often framed as a time of loss, but in reality, it is a time of deep awakening. It's a time to shed outdated beliefs and reclaim your power. It's an invitation to step fully into your next era as the radiant, magnetic woman you are meant to be. Each chapter will guide you in using this energy to navigate the shifts with confidence, grace and empowerment. You'll learn how to align your body, mind and spirit, so that rather than feeling like you are fading, you'll realise you are rising.

This is your time. This is your transformation. And the most powerful shift of all? It's already underway.

It's called menopause.

Let's take a closer look.

What Is Menopause and Why Does It Matter So Much?

Let's start with the basics, because knowledge is power.

The word "menopause" has Greek origins. Breaking it down, *mēn* means "month," linked to the lunar cycle, and *pausis* means "to stop."[2] So menopause quite literally means "the end of monthly cycles."

But this is far more than just the end of your period. This is the beginning of a powerful metamorphosis.

Menopause is a profound, life-defining transition. And here's why it matters so much: Menopause could span up to a third of your life, according to the largest-ever global study conducted on it to date, as published in BMC Public Health.[3]

Yes, a third of your life. That's decades.

Imagine spending that much time navigating changes to your body, mind and emotions without tools, support or a sense of purpose. That's not the future we're claiming. That's why you're here.

Menopause doesn't happen overnight. In fact, the shift often begins long before your final period, with perimenopause symptoms appearing as early as 8 to 10 years beforehand. For many women, the physical, mental and emotional toll can be overwhelming. That's exactly why this book exists: to guide you through it with clarity, confidence and grace.

So let's be practical. How can you make this transition smoother, more manageable and dare I say, transformative?

A woman in her power knows: Self-awareness is everything. One of the most effective tools? Tracking your symptoms. Noticing patterns. Listening to your body. By paying attention to what's really going on, you begin to reclaim agency over your experience.

Later in this chapter, I'll walk you through how to use your own Menopause Symptoms Tracker, which is a simple tool that can completely change how you understand your body and your needs.

But before we get there, I want to take you deeper. Because menopause is not just about hormones.

It's about energy.

One of the most beautiful ways to understand this is through Traditional Chinese Medicine.

Traditional Chinese Medicine (TCM)

What if you viewed menopause as a pattern to understand, rather than a problem to fix?

That's the invitation of Traditional Chinese Medicine (TCM). It offers a perspective that is ancient, holistic and beautifully attuned to the rhythms of a woman's life. It's also a view that resonates deeply with me.

I was born in Hong Kong and spent part of my childhood there. TCM wasn't considered an alternative. It was simply a way of life. My first true encounter with menopause came through my mother's experience while we were living there. Watching her navigate those changes, I became curious about how Eastern traditions approached this profound transition.

In TCM, the body is viewed as an ecosystem that is interconnected, dynamic and wise. Menopause isn't treated as a flaw to fix. It's treated as a shift in energy, a recalibration of your life force.

Ancient texts, such as the *Huangdi Neijing* (The Yellow Emperor's Classic of Medicine), written around 300 BC, describe the kidneys as the storehouse of life essence.[4] They are not just physical organs, but the roots of vitality. As kidney energy (or *Jing*) gently declines over time, menstruation slows and eventually ends. This can create imbalances in *yin* and *yang*, which are believed to cause familiar symptoms like hot flushes, night sweats or anxiety.

But here's what makes TCM so powerful: It doesn't isolate your symptoms from your story. It looks at the whole of you.

Your diet. Your emotions. Your sleep. Your stress. Your past. Your energy.

All of this matters because no two women experience menopause in the same way.

Your journey is yours and is shaped by your ancestry, habits, environment and resilience. Some women experience menopause as a soft unfolding. For others, it strikes like a storm, shaking the foundations of what once felt certain.

Menopause is not something happening to you; it's something awakening within you.

Yes, it's physical. But the transformation is also spiritual. When you begin to understand your body, honour your energy and meet yourself with curiosity rather than judgement - you reclaim your power.

This mirrors one of the core teachings in Buddhism: Life is a river, always flowing. Change is constant. When we cling to the riverbank, resisting what's moving, we struggle. But when we let go and allow ourselves to move with the current, we discover ease. Menopause is part of that current. A bend in the river's path. Not the end of vitality, but a deepening into it.

In this view, detachment doesn't mean disconnection. It's about releasing the need to control every wave and instead becoming more attuned to the flow. You learn to observe your body's changing patterns with curiosity, rather than fear.

To let go of the tight grip on how things "should" be, and instead ask, "What is this season inviting me to understand?"

Whether your path includes modern medicine, herbal remedies, acupuncture or all of the above, what matters most is agency. Choosing what supports you and releasing what doesn't.

Because at the centre of this journey is your mindset. And your mindset shapes everything.

A woman rooted in her feminine energy doesn't see menopause as a loss. She sees it as an initiation, a powerful passage into a more unapologetic version of herself.

The Seven-Year Cycles in TCM

In TCM, a woman's life is seen as unfolding in seven-year cycles.[5] These cycles help us understand how energy changes over time and why supporting your body before menopause is just as important as during and after.

The concepts of *Qi* (energy) and *Jing* (essence) are central. You're born with a finite amount of *Jing*, your deep life reserves. Over time, *Jing* is gradually depleted through life, work, stress and reproductive functions. While you can't regenerate *Jing*, you *can* protect and preserve it with rest, nourishment and emotional balance.

Here's how the stages of menopause are mapped through this lens:

From 28 to 35: The Fifth Cycle

You are at your peak vitality, though oestrogen slowly begins to decline. Balance is key at this stage, and it should be equal parts giving and receiving, as well as rest and action.

Potential symptoms: Skin paleness, early signs of muscle slackening and thinning hair

Wellness tips: Prioritise mental and physical self-care. Nourish yourself with rest, mindful movement and grounding foods.

Element: Earth

From 35 to 42: The Sixth Cycle

This is a preparation phase. *Yang* energy starts to decline as the body begins its journey towards menopause. TCM emphasises strengthening the five key organs: liver, heart, spleen, lungs and kidneys.

Potential symptoms: Early ageing signs such as wrinkles, greying hair and low energy

Wellness tips: Focus on maintaining emotional balance, improving sleep quality, maintaining skin hydration and adopting a nourishing, anti-inflammatory diet.

Element: Metal

From 42 to 48: The Seventh Cycle

Menopause begins to approach. This is a reflective stage where unresolved emotional patterns often surface. Stress, trauma and anxiety can intensify symptoms.

Potential symptoms: Hot flushes, mood swings, palpitations and disrupted sleep

Wellness tips: Slow down. Support your *Qi* with breathwork, acupuncture, journaling and time in nature.

Element: Metal

From 49 onwards: The Second Spring

This is true menopause, a stage of celebrated renewal. In TCM, it's known as the water phase, a time of deep wisdom and surrender. Life shifts from outward focus to inner nourishment.

Potential symptoms: Night sweats, joint aches, dryness and fatigue

Wellness tips: Nourish your *Jing*. Rest often. Eat warming, mineral-rich foods. Build rituals that restore your energy.

Element: Water

At this stage, something profound begins to happen. The energy you once gave so freely to others begins its sacred return. You begin tending to your own garden, listening, honouring and restoring. The call is no longer to keep up, but to come home.

We return to the river analogy, thinking of life like a river, ever-changing, always flowing. In youth, the current is fast and eager. But as it bends, it slows and deepens. It invites you to notice what's beneath the surface.

Menopause is not the river stopping. It's a shift in its rhythm.

In many Eastern philosophies, the greatest wisdom lies in non-resistance. This doesn't mean giving up. Rather, it's a release of the illusion of control. When we let go of the tight grip on who we used to be, we free up space to truly meet who we are becoming.

In this phase, you are becoming someone powerful. Someone rooted.

So as this cycle begins, I invite you to soften into it.

Let go of chasing.
Let go of overgiving.
Let go of needing to fix what was never broken.

Instead, begin asking:

What truly nourishes me now?

What is my body asking for that I've been too busy to hear?

Where can I begin again, and not as a version of who I was, but as the woman I am now?

Menopause is not your undoing. It is your becoming.

Let's keep flowing.

What Exactly Is Menopause in Modern Medicine?

Where TCM views menopause as an energetic transformation, modern Western medicine often defines it through biology, focusing on hormonal changes that occur over time.

According to the World Health Organisation (WHO), menopause is diagnosed after 12 consecutive months without menstruation.[6] The British Menopause Society reports that it typically occurs between the ages of 45 and 55, with the average age in the UK being 51.[7]

Biologically speaking, menopause marks the end of reproductive function. The ovaries stop releasing eggs and gradually produce less oestrogen, progesterone and testosterone. This shift can spark a wide range of changes, some subtle, others more dramatic. You might experience hot flushes, disrupted sleep, mood swings or changes to your skin, hair or libido. Some women hardly notice a thing. Others feel like strangers in their own bodies.

What's more, there's no specific starting point.

Perimenopause, which is the phase leading up to menopause, can begin in your late 30s or early 40s, and it doesn't always arrive with a clear signpost. It's different for every woman.

Take my mother's story. Her first signs weren't hot flushes, they were dry, dehydrated skin, skin tags, unexpected breakouts and a frozen shoulder. The flushes came later. For years, she was navigating perimenopause without even knowing it had started. Sound familiar?

Menopause isn't one moment in time. It's more similar to a journey. One that unfolds gradually, uniquely and often silently at first.

That's why awareness matters. It's about being prepared instead of scared. The more you understand what's happening in your body, the less confusing or isolating this transition feels.

Common Menopausal Symptoms

What makes menopause so fascinating – and frustrating – is that it shows up differently for everyone. Geography, culture, diet, stress and genetics all influence the intensity and variety of symptoms.

In a global study, data was gathered from over 480,000 middle-aged women during 2000-2023.[8] Hot flushes and night sweats topped the list of common symptoms, especially in the US, where up to 82% of women reported experiencing them. In Asia, the numbers ranged from 22% to 63%. These differences highlight the importance of personalised, culturally informed care.

Skin changes were another major finding, with around 50% of women reporting dry, itchy skin or a noticeable shift in texture and radiance. And yet, symptoms go far beyond the physical.

Let's break it down:

Physical symptoms: Changes in skin, bones, hair and joints. Oestrogen plays a crucial role in collagen production, so as levels fall, skin may become drier, thinner or more sensitive.

Psychological symptoms: Mood swings, anxiety, low self-esteem or a sense of emotional disconnection. These often go unspoken, but they are real, valid and deeply impactful.

Vasomotor symptoms: Hot flushes, night sweats and palpitations. These are linked to how oestrogen affects the brain's temperature regulation.

And these are just the headline symptoms.

You may also notice brain fog, fatigue or changes in digestion. Not every woman will experience all of these, but every symptom is worth paying attention to.

Because understanding what's happening gives you something incredibly powerful: agency.

You don't have to suffer in silence. You don't have to second-guess your experience. You don't have to just "get on with it."

This is your body's evolution, and you have every right to meet it with knowledge, compassion and support.

A more detailed but not exhaustive list of menopausal symptoms is as follows:

PHYSICAL	PSYCHOLOGICAL	VASOMOTOR (These relate to the body's heat regulation)
• Heart palpitations • Difficulty sleeping • Fatigue or lack of energy • Dizziness or fainting • Headaches • Tinnitus • Dry mouth and eyes • Sore gums • Muscle and joint pain • Breathing difficulties • Needing to urinate more often or experiencing leaks • Vaginal dryness or soreness • Increased thrush or cystitis • Dry or itchy skin • Thinning hair • Poor sleep	• Low mood • Anxiety or nervousness • Memory problems • Panic attacks • Difficulty concentrating • Loss of interest in most activities • Depression or feeling unhappy • Crying spells • Irritability • Mood swings • Loss of confidence • Reduced self-esteem • Brain fog • Loss of interest in sex or difficulty with arousal	• Hot flushes • Night sweats

These symptoms are referred to on the Menopause Charity website.[9]

Personalising Your Menopause Experience

Do any of these symptoms resonate with you?

For the purposes of this book, we're going to focus on two of the most common symptoms: hot flushes and skin changes. These were the symptoms my mum struggled with the most, and after speaking to other premenopausal and postmenopausal women, it's clear they're at the top of the list of issues most women would love more help with.

It's hard to predict exactly when perimenopause will begin for any woman. In my mum's case, she started showing early menopausal symptoms in her early 40s, long before she experienced her first hot flush at 46.

And the timing of those symptoms? Far from linear.

Some days and months passed seamlessly without any sign of change, while other times, symptoms like hot flushes lingered for years, coming and going unpredictably.

This is why it's so important to start tracking your symptoms. It helps you make sense of the menopause journey, allowing you to see patterns, identify triggers and gain a deeper understanding of what your body is going through.

A simple tracker can help you connect the dots and tailor your approach to managing the symptoms.

Here's an example of a populated tracker:

Date	Symptom	Possible Causes	How long did the symptom last?	What did I do to alleviate the symptom?	On a scale of 1-10 (1 low pain and 10 high pain), how painful is this symptom?
10 June 2025	Hot Flush	Feeling stressed and anxious while delivering a presentation and getting work done quickly before a client lunch It was a hot day, with temperatures of 25 degrees Celsius upwards	20 minutes in the afternoon	Deep breaths in the bathroom Changed into a strappy top Took a short walk to cool down	6 or 7 Was very uncomfortable

For quick access to the Menopause Symptoms Tracker, scan the QR code at the end of the book for exclusive access on https://shanti3.com/pages/book-form.

Tracking your symptoms and identifying patterns is an empowering process that puts you in the driver's seat of your menopause journey. By paying attention to possible causes like changes in your diet, sleep quality, hydration and emotional wellbeing, you can begin to understand how these factors might be influencing your symptoms. Even subtle shifts like weather, physical activity or how much time you've spent caring for others versus yourself can have an impact.

By consistently tracking, you can take proactive steps to alleviate symptoms. This process shifts your mindset from feeling like ageing is something that happens to you, to one where you actively shape how you navigate this life stage. The key is consistency; regular reflection helps you become more aware of your body's needs and what supports your vitality.

A woman rooted in her power knows her body is a temple – sacred, dynamic and ever-evolving. She doesn't retreat in the face of change; she listens, learns and adapts with grace. Even as her body shifts, she moves with the quiet authority of someone who has lived, loved and earned her wisdom.

She tracks her symptoms, not out of fear, but from deep respect. She observes, reflects and honours what her body is telling her. She understands that knowledge is power and that true self-care is an act of devotion.

If you're thinking, "I don't have time for a symptoms tracker," or if you're always on the go, just jot these headers into the Notes app on your phone. That way, you'll have a quick and easy record right at your fingertips.

A wise woman adapts. She follows through on her commitments to her wellbeing. She reclaims her story. She knows that tracking isn't about obsessing, it's about understanding. It's about recognising patterns, finding balance and making empowered choices that align with her body.

Many of the women I've spoken to, especially those in the midst of menopause, share a familiar story. They've spent decades putting everyone else first: partners, children, parents, work. Sound familiar?

The truth is, when you give so much of yourself away, it's easy to forget what you need. Especially now, when your body is asking you to listen more closely than ever before.

But here's what I want you to remember, and I can't emphasise this enough: Menopause is not the end of something. It's the beginning of a more intentional chapter. One where your needs rise to the surface. One where your voice matters most.

It's your moment to pause. To tend to yourself. To honour the woman you've become.

Think of it like the safety instructions on a plane: "Put on your oxygen mask first." Without doing that, how can you help anyone else?

Your wellbeing matters, not just to those around you, but to *you*.

This isn't selfish. It's essential.

I'll never forget talking to three beautiful women in their 60s and 70s at a wellness event. They approached me, curious about gua sha and skincare. One woman smiled and said, "I've never spent money on a skincare routine. I've always taken care of everyone else." I smiled and replied, "Aunty, it's never too late to start." We laughed together, and that stayed with me.

It's *never* too late to care for yourself.

Menopause is your opportunity. A call to turn inward with love.

Maybe your skin is changing. Maybe you're feeling waves of heat, sleep disruption or mood shifts. These aren't signs of something going wrong. They're signs your body is calling for attention.

Whether you're just stepping into this season or already walking through it, you're not simply enduring.

You're *rising*.

This phase of your life is not the closing act. It's a return to yourself, your strength and the deepest parts of your wisdom. You've made it this far with so much courage. And just as you've done before, you will move through this with grace.

But this time, it's for you.

Your body. Your rhythm. Your joy.

This is your next chapter.

Chapter 2
MENOPAUSAL SKIN

No matter how many years have passed, standing in front of the mirror and feeling like a stranger to your own reflection can be unsettling. But a goddess does not let a mirror define her. She does not scan for imperfections, nor does she measure her worth by the lines on her face. Instead, she sees what truly matters, which is how she *feels*.

The glow of wisdom in her eyes, the freckles that hold memories of laughter and the softness of her lips that have spoken words of love and strength. She understands that beauty is not something she is losing; it is something she has always carried within her.

Ageing is natural, yet it often catches us off guard. The changes happen gradually, almost imperceptibly, until suddenly they feel undeniable. And let's be honest, when you feel good in your skin, you move differently. You radiate confidence, a presence that others can't help but notice. But when you fixate on fine lines, sagging skin or dryness, it's easy to believe that's all anyone sees.

I've spoken to so many women who have felt this shift, who tell me:

"I don't recognise my face anymore; my skin feels so dry and itchy."
"Where did these jowls come from?"
"Why won't this double chin go away?"
"My face is sagging, and I'm losing collagen so fast."

But here's the truth: No one is analysing your reflection the way you are.

The world sees your energy, the way your eyes light up when you speak, the warmth of your smile and the way you carry yourself. *That is what makes you magnetic.*

I remember watching my mother go through this phase. She had always had smooth, radiant skin, but suddenly, everything felt different. Her skin was dry, irritated and unresponsive to the products she had trusted for years. She told me it felt as though she had lost something overnight. I saw her frustration, how it chipped away at her confidence, how it made her feel disconnected from herself.

So, we worked together – not just on skincare, but on something deeper. We worked on reclaiming her confidence, her connection to herself and her ability to see her own beauty beyond the changes. And that's what I want for you, too.

Menopause is not just a physical transition; it's an awakening. A chance to step into your power with renewed confidence and grace. Understanding the changes in your skin isn't about chasing youth; it's about nurturing yourself, honouring the woman you are becoming.

So when you look in the mirror, see yourself the way a goddess would. Not through the lens of what's changed, but through the light of everything you are: confident, empowered and radiant from within.

Understanding Menopausal Skin

When menopause begins, one of the first signs is often skin ageing. You may notice that your skin becomes thinner, wrinkles deepen and a sense of dryness settles in. The firm, elastic skin you're used to may start to feel looser and less resilient. This happens because oestrogen, a key hormone for skin health, starts to decline. With lower oestrogen levels, your skin produces less collagen and sebum (natural oils), which leads to dryness, sagging and a loss of that youthful glow.

During perimenopause – the years leading up to menopause – your hormone levels fluctuate. This can lead to a rollercoaster of skin issues, from oiliness one day to dryness the next. By the time you're in full menopause, sebum production has slowed significantly, leaving skin drier and more prone to itching. Thinning skin or skin atrophy becomes more noticeable due to rapid collagen loss.

In the first five years of menopause, women can lose up to 30% of their collagen, followed by a gradual decline of about 2% each year for the next decade and beyond.[10] That's a huge shift, and it can make skin appear drastically different from what you're used to.

Additionally, oestrogen influences melanin production, which is why you may notice your skin becoming lighter or more prone to age spots. These dark spots, often exacerbated by sun exposure, can appear more pronounced as your skin loses its ability to regenerate quickly.

The skin, as the largest organ of the body, is also the most exposed to the environment, especially areas like your face, neck, hands and arms. So while menopause is an internal transition, its effects on your skin are highly visible.

The good news is that understanding these changes can help you adapt your skincare routine to better support your skin's health through this phase of life.

10 Menopausal Skin Symptoms and What You Can Do About Them

Here are the 10 most common menopausal skin conditions, along with some practical tips for managing them.

Take what resonates with you, and leave the rest. If you know a friend, family member or colleague going through similar changes, feel free to share this with them. The more knowledge we have about menopausal skin, the better equipped we are to manage symptoms, feel confident and support our skin's natural healing.

No.	Skin Condition	What's Happening	Recommended Actions
1	**Dryness and Wrinkles**	Lower oestrogen levels lead to a decline in collagen production, reducing elasticity, which causes dry, thinning skin and an increase in wrinkles. Skin may appear dull and lose its youthful glow.	Look for moisturisers that contain hydrating ingredients like hyaluronic acid, glycerin or ceramides. In the evening, incorporate a facial oil into your routine for added nourishment. Try to avoid products with heavy fragrances and limit over-cleansing, as this can strip the skin of its natural moisture. Make sure to choose products specifically designed for dry skin. And don't forget to apply sunscreen every day to protect your skin from UV damage!

No.	Skin Condition	What's Happening	Recommended Actions
2	**Loss of Elasticity**	A reduction in oestrogen causes a decrease in collagen and elastin, leading to sagging and loose skin.	To combat loss of elasticity, opt for firming creams that contain ingredients such as peptides, antioxidants or retinol. You might also want to try non-invasive treatments or incorporate daily facial massages. Gua sha is a great tool for lifting, sculpting and draining excess fluid from your face. Consistent facial massage can work wonders to tone and rejuvenate your skin.
3	**Redness from Hot Flushes**	Hormonal fluctuations can cause sudden heat surges, resulting in flushed or reddened skin, particularly on the face, neck and chest.	During a hot flush, a quick spritz of cooling water spray can provide instant relief. It's helpful to avoid known triggers like spicy foods, alcohol and stress. Wear breathable fabrics (skip polyester!) and consider trying gua sha to gently soothe and cool the skin.

No.	Skin Condition	What's Happening	Recommended Actions
4	**Acne and Breakouts**	Hormonal imbalances increase sebum production, clogging pores and causing breakouts, even if you've always had clear skin.	Opt for gentle, non-comedogenic cleansers and moisturisers. These products are specifically formulated not to clog or block your pores. If you have acne-prone skin, look for ingredients like salicylic acid to help manage breakouts. A simple, natural tip: Use rosewater on a cotton pad twice daily to cool your skin and calm inflammation. It's a soothing, effective way to keep breakouts under control.
5	**Rosacea**	Hormonal shifts can trigger rosacea, causing redness, visible blood vessels and small, red bumps on the face.	Use skincare designed for sensitive skin and avoid harsh scrubs. Avoid washing your face with very hot or cold water; lukewarm is best. Rosewater is also a great option for calming inflammation. Applying it twice daily can make a significant difference.

No.	Skin Condition	What's Happening	Recommended Actions
6	**Prickly Skin (Weird Sensations)**	Declining oestrogen affects nerve endings, causing odd sensations like tingling, prickling or itching without a clear reason.	Those prickly, tingling sensations can be triggered by temperature extremes, so try to avoid overly hot or cold feet at night. When the tingling starts, use a cooling spray and moisturise regularly. Calming, anti-itch creams with ingredients such as aloe vera or colloidal oatmeal can also help soothe the skin. Choose soft, non-irritating fabrics and try taking a walk to boost circulation. Short walks can even help you sleep better.
7	**Facial Hair**	Hormonal imbalances, especially lower oestrogen compared to androgens, can cause unwanted facial hair growth, particularly on the chin or upper lip.	For smooth skin, consider hair removal methods such as waxing, threading or laser hair removal.

No.	Skin Condition	What's Happening	Recommended Actions
8	**Signs of Sun Damage**	Decreased oestrogen weakens the skin's natural protection against UV rays, making sun damage, such as age spots, hyperpigmentation and fine lines, more visible.	Make sunscreen your daily essential, especially SPF 50. I personally love Korean sunscreens as they're lightweight, don't leave a white cast and absorb beautifully into the skin. For an added glow, consider using brightening products with vitamin C and niacinamide to reduce sunspots and hyperpigmentation.
9	**Bruising, Fragile Skin and Slow Wound Healing**	Lower oestrogen levels can cause thinning of the skin, making it more prone to bruising, tearing and slower healing.	Use a daily moisturiser with ceramides to strengthen the skin. Avoid harsh treatments and protect your skin from injury.

No.	Skin Condition	What's Happening	Recommended Actions
10	**Jowls**	The loss of collagen and elastin due to lower oestrogen levels can result in sagging skin along the jawline, leading to the appearance of jowls.	As the skin loses elasticity, firming creams with peptides and antioxidants can help restore a youthful appearance. For a natural lift, use a gua sha to massage and sculpt your jawline. It can also help ease any tension you might be holding in that area.

My Mum's Skincare Routine for Dry, Menopausal Skin

When my mum started experiencing the most common menopausal skin issues – dryness and dehydration – I knew we had to create a skincare routine tailored to her changing needs. Below, I'm sharing her personalised regimen, designed specifically for dry skin. Please note that these are personal recommendations, not professional advice. Always seek guidance from a dermatologist if you have specific concerns.

If you experience irritation from a product, stop using it immediately. And remember, if you have sensitive skin, patch test any new products.

Time of day	Skincare Step	Why?
Morning	Wash skin with lukewarm water	Avoid extreme temperatures. Hot or cold water strips moisture from the skin.
Before and After Exercise (If Applicable)	Apply two to three drops of rosewater on a cotton pad and apply all over the face	Rosewater is anti-inflammatory and soothes redness while hydrating the skin.

Time of day	Skincare Step	Why?
During Shower	Use fragrance-free shower gel or soap and a fragrance-free shower oil	Whilst showering, apply a fragrance-free shower oil to damp skin and areas that require extra care, such as the arms, legs and chest. The shower oil absorbs more effectively when the skin is still warm and damp, helping to lock in moisture. Rinse off the shower oil with warm water. Be careful, as oils can make the tub or shower slippery.
Post-Shower	Apply two to three drops of rosewater on a cotton pad and apply all over the face	The benefits of rosewater are numerous. It's hydrating, anti-inflammatory, antibacterial, anti-ageing and balances your skin tone. Also, the cooling sensation feels nice!
Post-Shower	Apply Vitamin C serum	Vitamin C helps brighten the skin, boost collagen and protect from environmental damage.
Post-Shower	Layer with a fragrance-free, low comedogenic facial oil	Facial oils help lock in moisture, improve hydration and create a barrier to prevent water loss. They also help skin appear plumper and reduce fine lines.

Time of day	Skincare Step	Why?
Post-Shower	Apply SPF 50 sunscreen	Sunscreen is essential every single day. Korean sunscreens often have a lightweight, non-greasy formula that blends easily into the skin.
	Moisturiser	To seal in all the products and provide additional hydration.
Daytime	Top up SPF throughout the day, if needed	Protect your skin from UV damage throughout the day.
Evening	Remove makeup (if applicable) with micellar water and apply rosewater	Micellar water gently cleanses, and rosewater hydrates and soothes.
	Apply a couple of drops of hyaluronic acid serum	Hyaluronic acid is a humectant, which draws water to the skin. Applying it to damp skin helps increase absorption for deeper hydration.
	Layer with a fragrance-free, low comedogenic facial oil	This locks in moisture overnight, keeping the skin hydrated.

Time of day	Skincare Step	Why?
Evening	Gua sha routine	I'm obsessed with gua sha. It sculpts the jawline, lifts cheekbones and promotes lymphatic drainage to reduce puffiness and inflammation. Plus, it can help reduce wrinkles.
	Apply eye cream	The skin around your eyes is more delicate and prone to dryness, so a good eye cream can help reduce puffiness. Gently dab a pea-sized amount of eye cream around your orbital bone, tapping it in with your ring finger for light pressure.
	Use a thick moisturiser with beeswax	Beeswax locks in moisture, strengthens the skin barrier and protects against environmental stressors. It enhances elasticity and keeps the skin soft.

Why We Opted for a Natural Approach

Instead of jumping on the hormone replacement therapy (HRT) bandwagon to boost skin hydration and thickness, we decided to take a more natural route.

Here's why: About 10 years ago, my mum had a severe allergic reaction to Diclofenac, a common pain relief medication. I'll never forget the sound of a loud thud coming from the bathroom. I rushed in to find her unconscious on the floor, disoriented. Panicked, I immediately called for an ambulance. She was rushed to A&E and administered an EPIPen, which thankfully saved her life. After experiencing something so terrifying, I became a firm believer in trying natural remedies first before turning to medication. My mum feels the same way.

Ageing is a natural process, and for centuries, generations before us have relied on time-tested remedies.

In fact, one of the reasons I love rosewater so much is that it reminds me of my Nani, my grandmother. When I was little, I would watch my Nani place rosewater-soaked cotton pads on her eyelids before taking her daily 20-minute power nap. Even now, she still uses rosewater on her face with cotton pads. It's a natural ingredient that smells refreshing, is easily accessible and is incredibly affordable. My Nani has always had beautiful skin, and I believe that staying consistent with her skincare routine and relying on natural ingredients played a huge role in that.

For me, the goal is to heal the skin barrier and slow down the ageing process in a sustainable, long-term way, and of course, be a goddess. Quick fixes like Botox and fillers can be tempting, but they're not a lasting solution. Since women can spend up to 30% of their lives in menopause, it makes sense to focus on prevention, maintenance and healing when it comes to menopausal skin.

Skincare Tips and Tricks That Actually Work

No matter what skin condition you're dealing with during menopause, it's essential to start reading product labels. If a product contains fragrance, it's usually best to avoid it. The fewer chemicals, the better – your skin will thank you for it.

However, let's be real: Slathering on a bunch of skincare products and hoping for the best isn't going to magically fix everything. When it comes to ageing skin, especially during menopause, it's important to understand what's really going on. So, let's dive into the two main factors at play behind skin ageing: extrinsic factors (things you can control) and intrinsic factors (natural ageing that just happens).

Extrinsic Ageing: Environmental and Lifestyle Factors

This kind of ageing is caused by external factors, such as the sun, pollution and even lifestyle choices. The good news is that you have control here, and small changes can make a big difference.

Sun Exposure

You've probably heard it a thousand times, but it's true: The sun is the biggest culprit behind ageing skin. Excessive sun exposure can lead to wrinkles, dark spots and sagging skin.

Tip: Wear SPF 50 sunscreen every single day. Even if you're inside or it's cloudy, UV rays can sneak through windows. Make it part of your morning routine and don't forget to reapply during the day. Looking for something lightweight? Korean sunscreens are perfect for avoiding that dreaded white cast.

Pollution

Environmental pollution can damage our skin. It speeds up the appearance of wrinkles and dullness by attacking your skin with free radicals.

Tip: Start using an antioxidant serum (like Vitamin C) in the morning. Antioxidants neutralise those free radicals and help prevent skin damage, so think of it as a shield for your skin.

Smoking

Smoking doesn't just harm your lungs. It's also a fast track to losing collagen and elastin, leading to wrinkles, especially around your mouth.

Tip: If you're still smoking, quitting will not only improve your overall health but will also do wonders for your skin. Within weeks, you'll notice a brighter, healthier complexion.

Diet

Your skin reflects your lifestyle. Poor diet, lack of sleep and too much alcohol can lead to inflammation, dehydration and puffiness.

Tip: Fill your plate with antioxidants (berries, leafy greens and nuts) and healthy fats (avocados, salmon). Hydration is key, too. Drink plenty of water and limit your alcohol intake to keep your skin looking fresh.

Lifestyle Habits

Stress, lack of sleep and a hectic lifestyle all accelerate skin ageing.

Tip: Make sleep and stress management a priority. Try things like meditation, yoga or simply winding down with a good book and herbal tea at night. And remember, hydrate both inside and out!

Intrinsic Ageing: Natural, Biological Factors

Intrinsic ageing happens naturally over time, and it's mostly down to genetics. While you can't stop it completely, there are ways to manage it. Here's what's happening under the surface:

Loss of Collagen and Elastin

Collagen and elastin are proteins that give your skin its firmness and bounce. As we age, our skin's production slows down, leading to sagging and wrinkles.

Tip: Look for products that feature natural ingredients like plant-based oils (such as rosehip or argan) or antioxidants (like vitamin C). These can support collagen production and help keep your skin firm and supple.

Slower Skin Cell Turnover

As we age, skin cells don't renew as quickly, which can leave our complexion looking dull and uneven.

Tip: Use natural exfoliants, such as fruit enzymes from papaya or pineapple, once or twice a week, or opt for a water-based exfoliant. These gentle exfoliators can promote cell turnover and restore your skin's natural glow.

Loss of Subcutaneous Fat

The natural fat layer under your skin starts to thin out with age, which can lead to sagging.

Tip: Focus on using hyaluronic acid serums and thick moisturisers to plump up your skin and keep it looking fresh and hydrated.

Hormonal Changes

During menopause, your oestrogen levels drop, which makes your skin drier, thinner and more prone to irritation.

Tip: Moisturise like your life depends on it! Look for hydrating serums (hyaluronic acid, glycerin) and use a rich, fragrance-free moisturiser both day and night. Your skin will feel softer, more supple and less irritated.

How to Show Menopausal Skin Some Love

Stay hydrated. Dry skin is one of the most common issues during menopause, so focus on hydration. Use serums and moisturisers rich in ingredients like hyaluronic acid, ceramides and squalane. Natural oils, such as rosehip or jojoba oil, can also work wonders.

Embrace a gua sha routine. If you haven't hopped on the gua sha train yet, now's the time! It helps with lymphatic drainage, reduces puffiness and can even sculpt your jawline. Plus, it's a great way to relax.

Be gentle with exfoliation. While exfoliation is great for cell turnover, your skin can get more sensitive during menopause. Stick to gentle exfoliants instead of harsh scrubs.

Be consistent. No matter how good your products are, they need time to work. Be patient and stick with your routine. It's about long-term benefits, not instant results.

Prioritise rest and relaxation. Stress wreaks havoc on your skin, so make time for self-care. Whether it's through meditation, yoga or just relaxing with a cup of herbal tea, your skin will show the difference when you're less stressed.

Ageing is not something to fear. It is a rite of passage, a transformation, an initiation into a deeper, wiser, more powerful version of yourself. A goddess does not resist change; she embraces it, knowing that every phase of life brings new gifts. Menopause may shift your body, your skin and your energy, but it does not diminish your beauty. Instead, it reveals a new kind of radiance, one rooted in self-assurance, wisdom and the way you carry yourself.

Rather than chasing youth, nurture yourself. Build a skincare ritual that feels like an act of devotion, because that's exactly what it is. Protect your skin from the elements, nourish it with ingredients that support its changing needs and, most importantly, wear it with pride. The lines on your face are not flaws; they are stories, proof of a life well-lived, of laughter, love and resilience.

And remember, a goddess does not look in the mirror searching for what has faded. She sees what has *deepened*. She admires the glow of wisdom in her eyes, the strength in her features and the presence she commands without even trying. She does not apologise for time's touch upon her skin, because she knows that real beauty is not something that fades – it is something that grows.

If women spend a third of our lives in menopause, let us spend it in power, in joy and in confidence. Let us give our skin, our bodies and our souls the love and care they deserve.

Chapter 3
LET'S TALK ABOUT HOT FLUSHES

If you're navigating menopause, chances are you've felt the familiar rush of a hot flush at least once and probably many times over. Every woman I've spoken to on this journey brings up hot flushes, and it's no wonder. Hot flushes can strike out of nowhere, interrupting your day, breaking your sleep and leaving you feeling far from comfortable. But it's here where you can choose to shift your perspective. Navigating this is an opportunity to embody your divine feminine energy.

I see it every time I'm in class with my lovely Pilates ladies. Just before we hit the Pilates "hundred" (you know, that move that really makes you sweat), someone will always call out for the fan! And while we could all use the breeze during this exercise, for those going through menopause, it's almost essential.

Hot flushes were the exact reason I began researching a holistic approach to help my mum manage her menopause. It's one of the most challenging symptoms, showing up unannounced, bringing that intense, sudden warmth to your face, neck and chest, often followed by sweating, and sometimes even heart palpitations, headaches or feelings of faintness.

You're not alone in this. Over 88% of women experience hot flushes during menopause, with 50% of them living with this symptom for more than five years, and 10% experiencing it for more than 15 years, according to a study.[11] That's a long time to deal with these uninvited episodes! This is why shifting into a goddess mindset is everything.

What Is a Hot Flush?

In simple terms, it's a sudden, intense wave of warmth that spreads over your chest, neck and face, followed by sweating. They're often triggered by heat, hot drinks or even stress. Each episode can vary in length and intensity, from a brief few minutes to what feels like an endless cycle. As menopause progresses, the frequency and severity often increase, peaking about a year after your last period. The symptom may continue for months or even years after.

While each woman's experience is unique, the impact of hot flushes is undeniable. They don't just affect your body; they can disrupt your life and, most importantly, your wellbeing.

Understanding and Managing Your Hot Flush Triggers

Hot flushes can be incredibly troublesome, whether you're at home minding your own business or in the office, just about to head into a meeting. Why is it that a hot flush seems to creep up on you at the worst possible time? Suddenly, you feel that familiar wave of heat wash over you. Sound familiar? If you're experiencing this, you're definitely not alone. Each woman's journey through menopause is unique, yet many encounter similar triggers for hot flushes. Many women have found simple yet effective ways to manage and even minimise hot flushes. Understanding your triggers and making small adjustments can make a world of difference, helping you feel more in control.

Below, in another beautiful table, you'll find insights from real women who've discovered what works for them. If any of these ideas resonate with you, they're worth trying out. And stick around, because I saved the best tip for last!

No.	Topic	Why does it happen?	What has worked for others
1	Warm Environments	Hot flushes are often triggered by heat, whether it's from a warm room, direct sunlight or cosying up with heavy blankets.	Dressing in light, breathable layers that you can remove easily is a go-to trick. Many women recommend cotton or linen over synthetic fabrics, as they tend to trap heat. A portable fan can be a lifesaver, too; some women keep one in their bag or on their nightstand. Cooling sheets and a light blanket at night can also help you sleep more comfortably.

No.	Topic	Why does it happen?	What has worked for others
2	**Cold, Greasy and Spicy Foods**	Surprisingly, cold or raw foods can be harder to digest, making your body work harder and generating more heat. Spicy foods and heavy, greasy meals can also elevate your body temperature, often leading to flushing and sweating.	Many women find relief by focusing on warm, cooked meals, such as soups, stews and steamed vegetables. Switching to lukewarm drinks during the day, instead of icy cold ones, may also help. If you're a fan of spice, try gradually reducing it and note any changes. Using a Menopause Symptoms Tracker can help you identify patterns, making it easier to spot foods that tend to trigger flushes
3	**Alcohol and Caffeine**	Both alcohol and caffeine dilate blood vessels, which can intensify hot flushes. Red wine is a common trigger for many.	Many women find it helpful to limit their intake of coffee and alcohol, especially in the evenings. Herbal teas, like chamomile or chrysanthemum, which have cooling properties, make great alternatives. If you love the ritual of wine or cocktails, try non-alcoholic versions. One close friend swears by alcohol-free sparkling wine for the experience without the flush. If you're out at a pub or party, soda water with a splash of bitters and a slice of lime is a refreshing choice that's also great for digestion.

No.	Topic	Why does it happen?	What has worked for others
4	**Stress and Anxiety**	Stress hormones, such as adrenaline, can raise body temperature and often trigger a hot flush.	Practising deep breathing, meditation or gentle yoga can help calm the nervous system, which may reduce the intensity of flushes. Even taking five minutes each day for mindful breathing or gratitude journaling has made a difference for many women. Remember, self-care isn't selfish; it's essential, especially when it comes to managing stress-related flushes.
5	**Smoking**	Smoking affects blood vessels and hormone levels, making hot flushes more frequent and intense	Reducing or quitting smoking has had a profound impact on managing symptoms for many women. If quitting feels daunting, consider support groups, nicotine patches or consulting a healthcare provider for guidance. Some women have also found acupuncture helpful in managing cravings and reducing menopausal symptoms.

No.	Topic	Why does it happen?	What has worked for others
6	Exercise	Exercise raises body temperature, especially intense cardio workouts, which can lead to hot flushes during or after your routine.	Lower-intensity exercises, like yoga, Pilates or swimming, are easier on the body's temperature regulation. If you prefer more vigorous exercise, try exercising in a cool room or early in the morning. Weight training, a couple of times a week, is essential as the body loses bone density with age. Many women bring a cooling towel to the gym, which can be a quick way to lower body temperature. A refreshing shower after exercise can also help cool you down and prevent post-workout flushes.
7	Hormonal Fluctuations	During menopause, hormone levels naturally fluctuate, leading to unexpected hot flushes.	While you can't directly control hormone fluctuations, tracking patterns can be incredibly helpful. Using the Menopause Symptoms Tracker, you might find that flushes happen at certain times of the day or during specific activities. Recognising these patterns can help you adjust your schedule or environment to minimise discomfort.

No.	Topic	Why does it happen?	What has worked for others
8	**Tight Clothing**	Tight, non-breathable clothing can trap heat, making you more likely to experience a flush.	Opting for loose, breathable fabrics like cotton or linen can make a noticeable difference. Many women avoid layers or collars around the neck, where heat tends to accumulate. As a tip, always travel with an extra top. If you're wearing a jacket, opt for a short-sleeved top underneath.
9	**Large Meals and Sugar**	Eating large or carb-heavy meals can temporarily raise your metabolism, potentially triggering a flush.	Smaller, more frequent meals help maintain stable energy levels and prevent blood sugar spikes that could trigger flushes. Avoiding heavy, sugary meals, especially in the evening, may also improve the quality of your sleep. Whole, unprocessed foods tend to be gentler on the body and less likely to cause sudden temperature changes.

No.	Topic	Why does it happen?	What has worked for others
10	**Cold Glass of Water on the Wrists**	When you feel a hot flush coming on, cooling down specific pulse points on your wrists can help lower your overall body temperature.	Keeping a cold glass of water nearby and placing it on your wrists when a flush begins has been an instant fix for many women. The coolness on this sensitive area of the wrist helps bring down body temperature quickly. Whether you're at home or out and about, this small trick can make a big difference. It's subtle too, so you don't draw too much attention, perfect if you're in the office.
11	**20-Minute Nap for Energy**	Hot flushes and night sweats can sap your energy, leaving you feeling fatigued throughout the day.	A quick 20-minute power nap can be incredibly rejuvenating and helps you bounce back with more energy. This practice can especially be helpful if you experience disrupted sleep due to night sweats. Many women swear by this as a simple yet effective way to combat fatigue.

No.	Topic	Why does it happen?	What has worked for others
12	**Night Sweats**	Hot flushes during the night, also known as night sweats, can disrupt your sleep, leaving you feeling tired and irritable.	Here's the tip I saved for last because it's been a game-changer for so many: Try a warm foot soak before bed! Soaking your feet in warm water for about 20 minutes before bedtime can help regulate your body temperature. Warming your feet dilates blood vessels and releases heat from your body, lowering your core temperature so you're less likely to experience night sweats. To enhance your experience, add Epsom salts and a couple of drops of basil essential oil to the foot bath. Basil has an oestrogen-like compound that may help reduce the intensity of hot flushes. This simple, relaxing ritual has helped many women get a more restful night's sleep with fewer interruptions from night sweats

You're probably thinking that this all sounds easier said than done. Yes, these tips sound great on paper, but how do you actually implement them when the unpredictability of a hot flush can throw your day into chaos?

Mindset is everything when it comes to managing a hot flush.

A goddess knows that sudden waves of heat that rise from within, leaving you breathless, flushed and sometimes overwhelmed, are not a force to be feared or resisted. What if, instead of battling them, you saw them for what they truly are? A surge of energy, a transformation unfolding in real time? What if a hot flush was not something happening *to* you, but rather an invitation to pause, reflect and reconnect with yourself?

When you feel the warmth building, take a moment to check in with yourself. How are you feeling emotionally in this moment? Are you in need of more rest or self-care? Are you under stress? Just as a woman taps into her divine feminine power, moving through life with grace, poise and acceptance, you too can pause, breathe deeply and realign with your inner calm. Allow the hot flush to pass without resistance, knowing that it is temporary and your body is simply asking for a moment of attention.

Goddess Grounding Meditation for Hot Flushes

A goddess knows her body is sacred, wise and always evolving. She does not resist change. Instead, she flows with it, knowing that every transformation carries power. This meditation is your divine tool for navigating hot flushes with grace, balance and control.

For exclusive access to this meditation as an audio, scan the QR code in the conclusion or you can access through this link: https://shanti3.com/pages/book-form

Make this a ritual, a sacred practice, whether you do it in the morning to set the tone for your day or at night to invite deep, cooling rest.

Step 1: Find Your Sacred Space

Sit comfortably, with both feet planted firmly on the ground. Rest your hands gently on your lap, palms facing upward, open to receiving.

Close your eyes. Breathe in deeply, drawing in peace and clarity. Breathe out fully, releasing resistance, stress and discomfort.

Take three slow, deep breaths. Inhale through your nose. Exhale fully through your mouth. With each breath, let tension melt away.

Step 2: Visualise Healing Light

With your eyes closed and your breath steady, imagine a golden light flowing down from the universe. Picture it entering through the crown of your head, filling every inch of your body with warmth, safety and healing energy.

With every inhale, this light dissolves tension and discomfort.

With every exhale, feel yourself sinking deeper into peaceful stillness, open to your body's wisdom.

Silently affirm:

> *I allow myself to enter a deep state of relaxation. My body is safe. My body is wise. I surrender to this moment with grace and ease.*

Step 3: Acknowledge the Heat

Instead of resisting the hot flush, embrace it. See it as a surge of divine energy – your inner fire, your transformation. This is not happening *to* you but *for* you.

Silently repeat:

> *This heat is not my enemy. It is a message from my body, reminding me to pause, breathe and reset.*

Step 4: Ground Yourself

Imagine yourself as a radiant goddess standing barefoot on the sacred earth. Feel roots growing from the soles of your feet, anchoring you deeply into the ground, absorbing the earth's cooling, stabilising energy.

Now, draw that cooling energy upward:

Through your feet...

Up your legs...

Past your hips...

Rising through each energy centre, aligning and soothing any areas of disharmony.

Let this refreshing energy flow to any part of your body holding heat, all the way up to the crown of your head.

With each inhale, breathe in cooling energy.

With each exhale, release resistance.

Step 5: Release and Replace

In this relaxed state, let go of limiting beliefs. Imagine the golden light now surrounding you completely, forming a protective, empowering halo.

Mentally release any negative thoughts about menopause, ageing or hot flushes. See them lift away like dark clouds, dissolving into the universe – no longer yours to carry.

Replace them with these affirmations:

> I embrace this phase of life with strength and grace.
> Hot flushes do not control me – I move through them with ease.
> My body is wise, and I trust its rhythm.
> I radiate confidence, beauty, and power at every stage of life.

Feel these words sinking into every cell of your being.

Step 6: Cool, Calm, Empowered

Now, imagine a gentle, cooling energy flowing from your head down to your toes, like a refreshing waterfall washing over you.

Feel your body temperature stabilise. Feel your heartbeat steady. Let a deep, unshakable calm fill your entire being.

When you're ready, slowly open your eyes.

Wiggle your fingers and toes.

Return to your day with clarity, confidence and peace.

Remember, a divine feminine does not fear the fire; she understands it as part of her body's natural rhythm. Instead of letting it overwhelm her, she allows it to flow through her, fully aware that she is in control of how she responds. Whenever a hot flush arises, use this meditation to reset, realign and move forward with grace.

Each hot flush that arises is a chance to reset, to reconnect with your body and to embrace this natural transformation with the poise and strength of an empowered divine feminine. It will pass, just as all things do. In the meantime, you will prove to yourself just how resilient, empowered and graceful you truly are.

If your hot flushes are recurring, the key is understanding and addressing the root issues that fuel them and night sweats. Poor sleep is often the "straw that breaks the camel's back" for women going through menopause. When you're exhausted, everything feels more challenging, and it's harder to make choices that help you avoid triggers.

Let's imagine a different morning, one that sets you up for success.

You've just had a blissful seven to eight hours of deep, quality sleep. You feel refreshed, energised and ready to start your day without that dreaded brain fog. Without even thinking, you have the motivation to exercise, so you head to a yoga or Pilates class, leaving you feeling centred and accomplished.

Now, because you're well-rested, you might not feel the immediate pull for a morning caffeinated coffee or tea. Maybe you opt for a calming herbal tea or a cup of hot water with lemon instead. You've already made three healthier choices: good sleep, movement and a caffeine alternative – and all before breakfast.

With this foundation, your energy stays steady, your stress levels are lower, and you're making food choices that support your body rather than reaching for sugary snacks to get through the afternoon slump. Feeling rested, you're calmer, more focused and less reactive. And because you're already taking steps to support your body, a hot flush becomes less overwhelming if it does show up.

This is the mindset of a divine feminine who is fully in control of her wellbeing.

Managing hot flushes isn't about trying to prevent every single one. It's about creating a lifestyle that minimises their impact and empowers you to cope with them when they do happen. It's not about perfection, but about building resilience and learning to respond with calm and grace, no matter what.

However, I know that saying this is one thing, and actually living it is another, especially when insomnia strikes. You may wake up drenched in sweat at 2am, unable to fall back asleep, feeling frustrated and depleted. These sleepless nights can feel defeating, and they make it harder to focus on self-care the next day.

The good news is, even small changes can begin to shift things over time. Focusing on improving your sleep hygiene and creating a restful environment can make a world of difference.

Remember, you don't have to change everything overnight. Take it one step at a time, knowing that each choice you make is a step toward more restful nights and, in turn, fewer daytime hot flushes.

You are not alone in this. And even on the tougher days, be kind to yourself. Give yourself grace, and know that each small adjustment adds up. You have the power to create a life where you feel in control, not just of hot flushes, but of your overall wellbeing.

Step into your goddess energy. You've got this.

Seema's Story

During a Pilates class one afternoon, Seema called out with a laugh, "Please turn on the fan! I'm sweating!" Her energy made us all smile, but as the class wound down, I noticed the tiredness in her eyes. After class, I caught up with her. Seema, always warm and friendly, didn't shy away from sharing what was going on.

"It's these hot flushes," she sighed. "No matter what I do, I can't sleep. Last night, I had the aircon on so cold my husband was buried under two blankets – and he's still complaining about it!" Despite turning her bedroom into an Arctic zone, the night sweats persisted. She woke up drenched, exhausted and frustrated.

The sleepless nights weren't just draining her physically; they were affecting every part of her life. "I can't think straight at work," she confided. "I've been snapping at people over nothing, and I feel like I'm losing control. I don't even recognise myself sometimes." Her employer, noticing her struggle, offered her a week off. While she appreciated the gesture, Seema admitted, "A break isn't the solution. I need something that actually works."

That conversation resonated with the rest of the Pilates class. One by one, the women shared their own struggles with hot flushes and sleepless nights. Uma, another regular, offered a hopeful suggestion: "The days I come to Pilates, I sleep like a baby." This sparked a lively discussion about what helps – and what doesn't.

Although I'm not at the menopause stage yet, I couldn't help but join in, sharing gua sha techniques and holistic remedies I'd researched to help my mum and clients. By the end of the chat, the room was filled with laughter, shared stories and a sense of solidarity.

Inspired by the exchange, Seema left determined to try everything. Over the next few months, she experimented with different approaches. Some worked, some didn't, but she kept adjusting. Slowly but surely, she pieced together a routine that worked.

But what struck me most about Seema was her approach to it all. Despite the frustration, she refused to see menopause as something happening *to* her. She wasn't a victim of hot flushes; instead, she channelled her inner goddess. She accepted what was happening, listened to her body and took charge of finding a solution. She was determined, unshaken and ready to reclaim her wellbeing.

Seema's Mindset Shift and Hot Flush Remedies from the Pilates Ladies

Rather than dreading each hot flush, Seema began to see them differently. Instead of resisting or getting frustrated, she embraced them as a sign from her body – a gentle (or sometimes fiery!) reminder to pause, breathe and reconnect.

Each time a flush rose within her, instead of reacting with irritation, she took a deep breath and centred herself. She didn't see it as an interruption but rather a call to slow down, listen and care for herself.

She never let setbacks shake her. She adapted, refined and slowly built a routine that allowed her to navigate menopause with grace and confidence.

Her breakthrough came with the development of a mindful evening routine. She realised that stress from work and life often lingered in her thoughts, disrupting her sleep. By journaling each night, she could offload worries and create a to-do list for the next day, easing her mind. "I stopped feeling like I was forgetting something," she explained, "and that helped me relax." Lowering her stress levels before bed transformed her sleep quality.

Seema's journey is a testament to the power of embracing menopause as a transition, not a battle. She didn't try to control every symptom. She simply learned to move with them.

Here's a list that combines Seema's go-to solutions with tips from the other Pilates ladies. Take what resonates with you, leave what doesn't and share these ideas with anyone who might need them. No one should have to navigate menopause alone.

Create a Cool Bedroom Environment

Seema quickly realised that the temperature of her bedroom was the first battle to tackle. Through trial and error (and some heated negotiations with her husband!), she found that keeping the room at around 18°C was the sweet spot. Cooler temperatures reduced those middle-of-the-night wake-ups drenched in sweat, and she finally felt more stable and comfortable while sleeping.

The Pilates ladies also chimed in on bedding choices, which turned out to be a game changer for many. Heavy blankets were swapped out for lightweight duvets, and cooling pillows became the new must-have. Natural fabrics, such as cotton, bamboo and linen, have earned rave reviews for their ability to regulate temperature, unlike synthetic materials that tend to trap heat.

Not everyone has air-conditioning, and that's okay. The ladies shared simple alternatives like keeping a small fan running or cracking a window when the weather allowed. Good airflow worked wonders to keep them cool and comfortable throughout the night.

Night-Time Hydration Strategy

Hydration seems like a no-brainer, but Seema learned the hard way that drinking too much water before bed could backfire. Not only did it lead to more frequent bathroom trips, but it also seemed to trigger her night sweats. Her solution? Spreading her water intake evenly throughout the day and taking just a small sip before bed if she felt thirsty.

She also swore by her evening herbal tea ritual. About two hours before bedtime, she'd settle down with a small cup of chamomile or chrysanthemum tea, which helped calm her mind and body. Cutting out caffeine entirely (or at least avoiding it after lunch) was another non-negotiable for her, as even small amounts seemed to disrupt her sleep.

Adopt a Mindful Evening Routine

Seema found that her stress levels were a major factor in her night sweats. The endless to-do lists and lingering worries from the day often followed her to bed, making it hard to wind down. That's when she started journaling in the evening. Writing down her thoughts and making a quick to-do list for the next day helped her feel lighter and more organised. "I stopped worrying that I was forgetting something," she said, "and that alone helped me relax."

Avoiding triggers became another focus. She steered clear of caffeine after lunch and cut back on alcohol and spicy foods, especially at dinner. These small adjustments noticeably reduced her night sweats.

Relaxation techniques, such as the 4-7-8 breathing method, became a nightly habit. Seema found this breathing technique decreased anxiety, increased her sleep quality, managed food cravings and controlled emotional responses, such as anger and frustration. Spending just a few minutes on deep, focused breathing helped her shift into a calmer, more restful state before sleep.

4-7-8 Breathing

1. Find somewhere comfortable to sit and close your eyes, if possible.

2. Close your mouth and inhale through your nose for 4 seconds.

3. Hold your breath for 7 seconds before you exhale.

4. Exhale slowly for 8 seconds.

Repeat steps 2 through 4 for a minimum of 5 repetitions.

I've been using this technique for years whenever I feel stressed, anxious or frustrated. It can be done anywhere and takes just 5 minutes to calm your heart rate and nervous system down.

Stick to a Consistent Sleep Schedule

This one sparked a debate among the Pilates ladies! Some, like Seema, found that going to bed and waking up at the same time every day, even on weekends, worked wonders for their sleep. Sticking to a routine seemed to help her body settle into a natural rhythm, which in turn improved both the quality of her sleep and the frequency of her night sweats.

Others firmly defended their weekend lie-ins, arguing that flexibility was key to their overall wellbeing. My takeaway? Listen to your body and find what works for you.

Light Movement and Stretching

Exercise was a game-changer for sleep management, a sentiment the Pilates ladies unanimously agreed on. However, timing and intensity made all the difference. Intense evening workouts were a no-go since they often left the body overheated and restless. Instead, gentle stretches or a relaxing Pilates session earlier in the day became the go-to for unwinding and releasing muscle tension.

Incorporating daily movement, whether it was a brisk walk, light cardio or a Pilates class, helped maintain balanced energy levels throughout the day. For many, this balance translated directly into deeper, more restorative sleep at night.

Cooling Sleepwear and Pre-Bed Foot Soak

Seema discovered that her choice of sleepwear was a surprisingly important factor. She swapped out her usual attire for loose, breathable pyjamas made from natural fibres like cotton. These lightweight fabrics helped her stay cooler and more comfortable, making a big difference in her night sweats.

One unique tip I shared with the Pilates ladies was to soak their feet in warm water for 20 minutes, about an hour before bedtime. It might sound counterintuitive, but this ritual actually lowers the body's core temperature by encouraging heat to dissipate through the feet. For Seema, this became a soothing pre-bedtime habit that signalled her body to relax and prepare for restful sleep.

Screen-Free and Low-Light Environment

Seema realised that her evening screen time was sabotaging her sleep. Blue light from phones, laptops and TVs interferes with melatonin production, making it harder to fall asleep. She made it a rule to turn off screens at least an hour before bed, opting instead for calming activities like reading or journaling. To complement this, she dimmed the lights in her home as bedtime approached, creating a serene, low-light environment that supported her body's natural sleep rhythm.

When it came to her bedroom setup, Seema invested in blackout curtains to block out any light and relied on earplugs to drown out nighttime noises, especially her husband's occasional snoring! These small adjustments turned her bedroom into a true sleep sanctuary.

Mindset and Patience

The most transformative part of Seema's journey was her mindset shift. She learned that stressing about her night sweats only made them worse. Instead, she approached her sleep challenges with patience and curiosity, experimenting with different strategies until she found the ones that worked best for her.

By focusing on what she could control and staying positive, Seema gradually reclaimed her nights and her energy. Her story is a powerful reminder that small, consistent changes – paired with a little perseverance – can lead to big improvements in sleep and overall wellbeing.

Seema's story is a beautiful example of stepping into divine feminine energy during menopause. She refused to let hot flushes control her. She listened to her body, adjusted her approach and found a way to thrive rather than just cope.

This is the power of the goddess mindset. Again, menopause isn't something that happens *to* you; it's a transformation that calls for grace, wisdom and self-care. It's a time to honour yourself, to trust in your resilience and to embrace every challenge as a reminder of your strength.

Like Seema, you too can navigate this transition with confidence, wisdom and poise. With the right tools, mindset and support, you can reclaim your balance, rest deeply and navigate menopause like the radiant goddess you are.

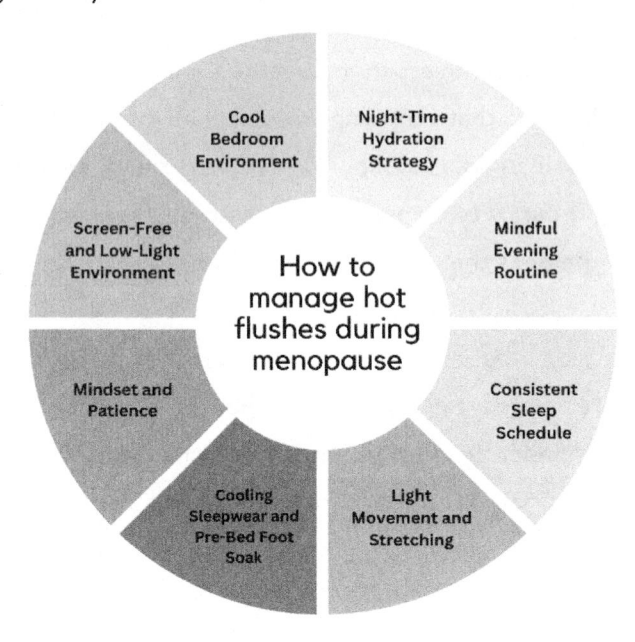

How to manage hot flushes during menopause:
- Cool Bedroom Environment
- Night-Time Hydration Strategy
- Mindful Evening Routine
- Consistent Sleep Schedule
- Light Movement and Stretching
- Cooling Sleepwear and Pre-Bed Foot Soak
- Mindset and Patience
- Screen-Free and Low-Light Environment

Shatavari for Menopause

Let's face it, dealing with hot flushes can feel overwhelming, especially when solutions feel out of reach. But sometimes, a simple, holistic remedy can make a world of difference.

I discovered this first-hand with my mum, who was grappling with intense hot flushes and wanted a natural solution. After diving into research, we discovered Shatavari, a herb deeply rooted in Ayurvedic tradition. While it wasn't mainstream back then, it's gaining traction now as more modern medical research highlights its benefits for menopausal women.

If you're exploring holistic ways to manage menopause, Shatavari could be a worthwhile option, especially if HRT isn't suitable for you or if you're concerned about the potential side effects, such as increased risks of breast cancer or heart disease. Here's why Shatavari has worked for many women, and why it might work for you, too.

What Is Shatavari?

For those new to it, Shatavari is a type of asparagus (scientifically known as *Asparagus racemosus*) cultivated in parts of India, Africa, Sri Lanka and China. Shatavari has traditionally been used for women's health across various stages of life, particularly during menopause. Shatavari is recognised as a powerful adaptogen and phytoestrogen, which means it can help the body manage stress and naturally balance hormone levels.

How Does Shatavari Work?

One of the main reasons Shatavari is beneficial for menopausal women is its high content of phytoestrogens or plant compounds that mimic oestrogen in the body. As oestrogen levels drop during menopause, it's often this lack of oestrogen that triggers hot flushes, night sweats, mood changes and other symptoms. The phytoestrogens in Shatavari act like mild oestrogen in the body by attaching to estrogen receptors. This gentle effect can help reduce menopausal symptoms naturally.

In addition to hormonal support, Shatavari's adaptogenic properties help the body manage stress. Stress is a major trigger for hot flushes, and reducing stress levels can help make menopausal symptoms more manageable. This combination, which supports oestrogen balance and reduces stress, makes Shatavari particularly effective.

What the Research Says

While Shatavari has been used in traditional medicine for centuries, scientific research is now validating these benefits. A recent study presented a case series involving 70 menopausal women aged 40 to 65.[12] Half of the group took a placebo, while the other half took 250 mg of Shatavari twice daily for eight weeks.

The findings? Women taking Shatavari experienced:

Fewer hot flushes. Both the frequency and severity of hot flushes were reduced.

Improved mood and reduced anxiety. Feelings of nervousness, irritability and anxiety decreased significantly.

Better sleep quality. Insomnia and night awakenings were less common, helping these women feel more rested.

Enhanced relationships. Improved mental wellbeing and reduced emotional swings helped many women report better relationships and social interactions.

Reduced vaginal dryness and **improved sexual wellbeing**. Hormonal balance improvements seemed to benefit intimacy and comfort.

This research offers scientific support for the traditional use of Shatavari, showing that it may help menopausal women manage a broad range of symptoms without the risks associated with synthetic hormone replacement.

When my mum started using Shatavari, it wasn't just a relief; it was a game-changer. Without HRT, she was relying solely on holistic remedies, and Shatavari quickly became her go-to. After a few weeks, she was experiencing fewer hot flushes, less intense night sweats and better overall mood stability. She felt more in control, which had a positive effect on her confidence and quality of life.

Seeing how effective it was, my mum recommended Shatavari to some of her friends who were also dealing with hot flushes. They too found that it helped reduce the severity of their symptoms and gave them a much-needed sense of relief and control. Each of them reported that the herb had become a regular part of their wellness routine.

Finding What Works for You

There is no one-size-fits-all approach to menopause. Each woman walks her own sacred path. But what remains constant is your inner power, your ability to flow with these changes rather than fight them.

If you're open to natural support, Shatavari may be a divine ally, helping to restore balance and nurture your body through this transformation. Keep a Menopause Symptoms Tracker, not just as a log, but as a sacred journal of self-discovery, revealing the rhythms of your body and what truly supports your wellbeing.

Take inspiration from Seema, who tapped into her goddess energy to move through hot flushes with ease, crafting daily rituals that soothed her body and honoured her needs. Whether it's mindful movement, cooling bedtime practices or tuning into the breath, your intuition will guide you to what resonates.

Now is the time to fully embody your divine energy. Rather than resisting the fire, welcome it. Each hot flush can be seen as a surge of inner power, a symbol of your transformation. Let it ground you, awaken you and reconnect you to your body's wisdom.

You are not at war with yourself. You are evolving, rising, becoming even more powerful. Claim this journey with grace, confidence and the deep knowing that you are truly unstoppable.

Part 2

ALL ABOUT GUA SHA

Chapter 4

AWAKEN YOUR INNER GODDESS WITH GUA SHA

Have you heard of gua sha? If not, don't worry. You're exactly where you need to be. This ancient, sacred skincare practice is far more than just a beauty technique; it is a ritual of self-love, renewal and empowerment.

Though I am not personally navigating menopause, my journey with gua sha began out of curiosity. What I discovered was something far deeper than skincare. Gua sha is a practice that connects you with your body, calms your mind and helps you move through transitions gracefully. For women in menopause, this practice becomes even more powerful, offering relief from dryness, sagging and the skin texture shifts that come with hormonal changes.

But gua sha is not just about appearances; it's about activating your goddess energy, embracing your evolving beauty and honouring your body's transformation. With every slow, intentional stroke, you move stagnant energy, increase circulation and reconnect with yourself in the most loving way.

In this chapter, we'll explore the magic of gua sha – what it is, how it works and why it is a game changer for menopausal skin. By the end, you will feel confident, radiant and ready to make this ritual your own.

What Is Gua Sha?

If you've never heard of gua sha before, let me explain. Gua sha (pronounced "gwa sha") is a healing technique that's been used for centuries in TCM. It's a therapeutic practice designed to restore balance, improve circulation and support overall health and vitality.

The word *gua* translates to "scrape" or "scratch", though it's worth clarifying that there's no harshness or abrasion involved. Instead, *gua* refers to the use of a smooth-edged tool to press and stroke lubricated areas of the skin in a deliberate and soothing manner. The term *sha* translates to "sand" or a fine, red rash-like appearance. This refers to the temporary redness that can appear on the skin after a session, signalling improved blood flow and the release of tension or energy blockages.

Far from being harsh, gua sha is a deeply rejuvenating process. It helps awaken your body's natural healing mechanisms, leaving you feeling refreshed and balanced inside and out.

What makes gua sha unique compared to other therapies is its focus on three key principles:

1. **Unidirectional stroking**. Gua sha technique involves firm, repeated strokes in a single direction to target the fascia (the connective tissue beneath the skin).

2. **Muscle line focus**. Unlike massages that may move across muscles, gua sha works along muscle lines to improve blood flow and release tension.

3. **Purposeful redness (Sha)**. The process intentionally creates light redness or "petechiae" on the skin, indicating that circulation and healing responses have been activated.

This redness is temporary but signifies that gua sha is doing its job, helping your body release blockages and promote recovery.

But before we explore further, let me share my journey and how I discovered the power of gua sha.

My Personal Story

Let me share something deeply personal, a time when my overall wellbeing hit a breaking point and I went through a mini existential crisis. It was one of those moments when life feels so overwhelming that your body starts screaming for attention and you don't know what to do. For me, that wake-up call came through my skin.

During the COVID lockdown, I was in the thick of it, working long hours as a structured finance paralegal in a U.S. law firm. Imagine 70+ hour weeks, back-to-back deadlines and the kind of stress that keeps you up at night. It was a relentless cycle of work, eat, minimal sleep, repeat. The days blurred together. Then, one morning, I woke up and stared at myself in the mirror, horrified. My face and body were covered in an itchy, red, angry rash. It looked like chickenpox. My skin was inflamed and uncomfortable. I couldn't stop crying.

I panicked. "How am I supposed to work like this? How do I attend meetings on a Zoom call?" I asked myself. "What if this is permanent? What if it left scars?"

But with a big deal closing the next day, I didn't even have time to process the rash and all the discomfort that came with it. That day, I managed to power through work, keeping my camera off during calls, all while feeling miserable in my own skin.

Later, I rushed to a GP (short for a "general practitioner" doctor in the UK), hoping for answers. But all I got was: "We can't be sure how this rash started... Keep it moisturised, and it'll heal on its own." The doctor offered me a steroid cream, but I refused. Deep down, I knew this wasn't something I could fix with a quick prescription. I needed to understand what was really going on.

The Turning Point

I was beyond frustrated. None of my usual skincare products were usable anymore. They either stung my irritated skin or were filled with hidden fragrances that only worsened things. I turned to an aqueous cream (a simple, baby-safe moisturiser) and slathered it on for two weeks. Slowly, the rash calmed down. The itching stopped, but redness and some spots lingered, and I lived in fear it might all come back.

Looking back, I believe it was my body screaming at me to slow down. Stress had wreaked havoc, not just on my skin, body and mental health, but also on my hair – I was losing it by the handful.

That's when my curiosity about natural healing kicked in. In all areas, I was researching spirituality, therapy and gentle, holistic ways to support my skin. That's how I discovered gua sha.

The Discovery

At first, I didn't know what to make of it. Sounds great in theory. Gua sha looked so simple. You just move a smooth stone tool to massage the skin in specific motions.

I thought to myself, *Could it really work? Is it effective? Will it heal my skin?*

Although slightly sceptical, what caught my attention wasn't just the technique, it was the philosophy behind it.

Gua sha isn't about quick fixes. It's about working with your body, not against it. Instead of trying to "fix" my skin, I saw gua sha as a way to support it, helping it heal, restore balance and function the way it was meant to.

Once my skin was calm enough to tolerate touch, I decided to give it a try.

My Gua Sha Ritual

Each morning, before the world demanded my attention, I carved out sacred time for myself, just five or ten minutes dedicated to my skin, my wellbeing and my inner goddess. I didn't see it as a beauty routine; for me, it was a ritual of self-love and renewal, a moment to honour my body and its changing rhythms.

I would take my gua sha tool in hand, apply a nourishing facial oil and begin the slow, intentional strokes I had learned. With each movement, I was lifting and sculpting my skin, and at the same time, I was awakening my divine feminine energy, reconnecting with my body and allowing stagnant emotions to melt away.

At first, it was simply a soothing practice, a small luxury in the midst of life's chaos. But as the days passed, something shifted. My skin became firmer, smoother and more radiant. The lingering redness faded. And more importantly, I felt deeply connected to my health, to my body and to myself.

That's when I made myself a promise to stop sidelining my wellbeing. A woman rooted in her power does not neglect herself. She honours her needs, embraces her beauty and tends to her body like the sacred vessel it is.

The Healing Power of Gua Sha

Gua sha is more than skin-deep; it is a tool of transformation and healing, aligning perfectly with the wisdom of TCM.

There is a saying in TCM:

"First treat the exterior, then the interior."

This means that by addressing imbalances on the surface, we prevent them from manifesting as deeper, more chronic issues.

Gua sha embodies this principle beautifully. It releases trapped heat, reduces inflammation and restores balance, not just in your skin, but throughout your entire system. After each session, I could see the difference: redness faded, puffiness reduced and my face was glowing with newfound vitality. In TCM, this is the power of moving stagnant energy, removing blockages, improving circulation and allowing the body's natural healing abilities to shine through.

But beyond the physical, this ritual is a reminder, a sacred pause to honour our evolving beauty and embrace the transformation happening within. With each stroke, we reconnect to our strength, radiate confidence and step into the full force of our feminine power.

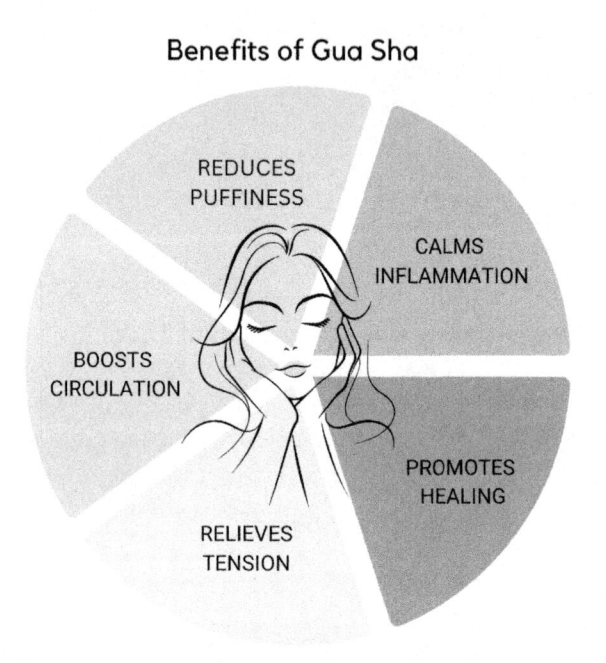

Benefits of Gua Sha

- REDUCES PUFFINESS
- CALMS INFLAMMATION
- PROMOTES HEALING
- RELIEVES TENSION
- BOOSTS CIRCULATION

Why Gua Sha Worked for Me

Gua sha is a transformative practice that helped me heal both physically and emotionally.

Here's what makes it so powerful:

Boosts circulation. Imagine giving your skin a workout. Gua sha increases blood flow, delivering oxygen and nutrients to your skin cells while flushing out toxins.

Calms inflammation. If you've ever dealt with redness, puffiness or discomfort, gua sha is like a gentle reset. By addressing stagnant energy (what TCM calls "stuck Qi"), it soothes inflamed areas and restores balance.

Reduces puffiness. Hormonal shifts, stress or even just a poor night's sleep can lead to fluid retention. Gua sha helps move those trapped fluids, leaving your skin feeling lighter and looking more sculpted.

Promotes healing. Gua sha stimulates your body's natural ability to renew itself. It encourages fresh blood flow, supports the creation of new cells and helps your skin recover from issues like irritation or dullness.

Relieves tension. We carry so much stress in our faces – tight jaws, furrowed brows, clenched muscles. Gua sha gently releases this tension, smoothing lines and helping you feel deeply relaxed.

Simply put, gua sha works by getting rid of what's stuck, calming what's inflamed and supporting your body's natural healing processes. As you can see, these benefits are particularly effective for changes to menopausal skin on the face and body.

As TCM teaches, when function is slowed or substances are stuck, pain and discomfort follow. Gua sha steps in to resolve that stagnation, bringing relief and restoring balance. Whether you're dealing with visible skin concerns, stress or deeper imbalances, gua sha is a powerful tool to help your body heal and thrive.

How Gua Sha Can Help You

No matter what you're going through, gua sha is a tool that meets you where you are.

For menopausal women: Hot flushes? Gua sha helps vent heat from your body, offering relief and cooling you down naturally.

For stressed and busy women: Whether it's fluid retention, jaw tension or that "heavy" feeling in your face, gua sha gives you a quick moment to reset and refresh.

For anyone feeling stuck: If you're battling puffiness, dull skin or just need to feel more grounded, gua sha works by moving what's stagnant, bringing you back to balance.

It's more than a beauty ritual; it's a way to reconnect with yourself, relieve stress and support your body's natural healing processes.

How Gua Sha Works Its Magic During Menopause

Menopause often feels like a whirlwind of changes, especially when it comes to our skin. Dryness, dullness and sagging are common concerns that can leave you feeling disconnected from the radiant, confident version of yourself. These changes are mostly due to declining oestrogen levels, which slow down collagen production and weaken the skin's barrier. Add to that a reduction in cell turnover, and it's no wonder your complexion can feel dehydrated, lacklustre or just plain tired.

This is where gua sha steps in as a natural, accessible tool that can make a world of difference. By integrating it into your routine, you can naturally address many of the challenges that menopause brings. Here's how gua sha supports you through menopausal symptoms:

Boosts Circulation for Better Hydration and Radiance

The intentional, pressed strokes of gua sha stimulate blood flow to the skin, improving oxygen and nutrient delivery. This enhanced circulation helps replenish the skin's hydration levels, which are often depleted during menopause. With consistent use, your complexion will look more radiant, plump and refreshed.

Promotes Lymphatic Drainage to Reduce Puffiness

Gua sha is highly effective in stimulating the lymphatic system, which is responsible for removing toxins and excess fluid. During menopause, your lymphatic system slows down (a common occurrence with age), which can lead to puffiness and a tired appearance, especially under the eyes. Gua sha helps get the lymphatic fluid moving, flushing out toxins and reducing swelling. The result? A firmer, more sculpted appearance.

Restores Collagen for Firmer Skin

Collagen loss during menopause can make skin sag and fine lines more pronounced. Gua sha stimulates collagen production by increasing circulation in the deeper layers of the skin. This helps lift and firm areas like your jawline, cheeks and forehead, giving your face a naturally lifted look.

Encourages Cell Turnover

Although gua sha isn't a traditional exfoliator, its ability to improve circulation encourages fresh, healthy skin cells to rise to the surface. This can smooth out rough patches, soften fine lines and enhance overall texture.

Supports Hydration and Skin Barrier Repair

When used with a hydrating serum or facial oil, gua sha allows the product to penetrate more deeply into the skin. This not only enhances hydration but also strengthens your skin's barrier, helping it retain moisture longer and combat menopausal dryness.

Releases Tension for a Relaxed, Youthful Look

Menopause can be stressful, and stress shows up on your face as tension. Gua sha's soothing motions help release tightness in your facial muscles, smoothing expression lines and leaving you with a softer, more relaxed appearance.

I'm often asked, "How do I fix this? How do I get rid of puffy under-eyes, lift my jawline or deal with dryness?" Time and time again, I tell women there's a gua sha solution. Let me share more about how it can work for you and how it's already transformed lives.

Why I Believe in Rituals, Not Quick Fixes

These days, it feels like we live in a world of instant gratification. Botox, fillers and lasers; they promise immediate results, but they don't address the root cause. The underlying issues – stress, inflammation, hormonal changes – are still there, bubbling under the surface.

Gua sha taught me the value of slowing down and listening to my skin. Ageing is a natural process, and our skin is always communicating with us. When we tune in, we can address the root causes of our concerns and truly heal, not just "fix" the symptoms.

A Client's Story: From Pain and Puffiness to Relief and Radiance

One of my most memorable clients was a woman named Anna who came to me with a mix of physical discomfort and skin concerns. She'd been struggling with deep facial puffiness, sagging skin and dark under-eye circles that no amount of concealer could hide. She was also carrying years of tension in her upper back and shoulders, which was a chronic pain she chalked up to stress and posture.

Anna admitted she felt stuck. Menopause had left her body feeling foreign, and her confidence was at an all-time low. Traditional massages hadn't helped her shoulder pain, and expensive skincare routines had done little to restore her glow. I suggested trying gua sha, not just for her face but for her entire body.

We began with her face, working with gentle, rhythmic strokes along her cheekbones, jawline and under-eye area. Almost immediately, her skin started to look brighter, and the puffiness began to drain away. As I continued the session, Anna remarked that the gentle movements felt deeply relaxing, like a release she hadn't realised she needed.

Next, we moved to her body. Anna had a persistent knot in her upper left shoulder that had troubled her for years. Using the pointed end of the gua sha tool, I began with firm, sweeping strokes to target the tension. The skin around the knot turned red, a sign of increased blood flow and movement of stagnant energy, which is a hallmark of the gua sha process. As we worked deeper into the area, the redness started to shift downward, and Anna let out a deep sigh. For the first time in ages, she felt relief.

As I worked on her body, I noticed poor circulation in her legs. Her right leg felt cooler to the touch, indicating lymphatic stagnation. Starting from her upper thigh, I used long, upward strokes down to her ankle, focusing on pressure points to encourage blood flow. By the end of the session, her right leg was noticeably warmer, and she could feel the difference in how her body moved. Without me even prompting her, Anna mentioned that her chronic knee pain had started to ease.

Over the next few weeks, Anna began practising gua sha at home, incorporating it into her nightly routine. She used a facial oil to enhance the tool's glide and worked on her face for just five or ten minutes each evening. For her body, she spent extra time on her shoulders and legs, focusing on the areas we'd worked on during her session. Slowly but surely, her skin regained its hydration and glow. The dark circles faded, her jawline became more defined and she felt lighter – not just physically, but emotionally, too.

It's More Than Skincare; It's a Goddess Ritual

What Anna discovered – and what I hope you will, too – is that gua sha is more than a skincare tool. It is a sacred ritual, a moment to reconnect with your body, honour your beauty and embrace your divine feminine power.

The best part? Gua sha is simple, affordable and easy to weave into your daily life. All it takes is consistency, just a few minutes a day to invest in yourself. Just as regular exercise strengthens your muscles and boosts your mood, regular gua sha strengthens your skin, relieves tension and restores balance to your entire being. It's a practice of devotion to yourself, a reminder that your wellbeing is worthy of time and care.

Let's put the myth to rest that skincare must be complicated or expensive. With gua sha, you're not just caring for your skin, you're also nurturing your whole self. It's a small step with profound rewards.

Reclaiming Your Power

For me, gua sha was more than just a beauty ritual. It was a way to reclaim my power in a time of chaos. It gave me the space to pause, to listen to my body and to heal – not just on the surface, but in a way that felt deeply personal and meaningful.

So, if you're feeling stressed, overwhelmed or disconnected from yourself, I can't recommend gua sha enough. The technique isn't about chasing perfection. Instead, it's about embracing your natural beauty, your transformation, and your inner strength.

In a world that moves too fast, gua sha invites you to slow down, to honour your body's wisdom and to give yourself the love and care you deserve. Because you, goddess, are worthy of that moment of devotion.

Chapter 5

GUA SHA TECHNIQUES

I'm honoured to guide you through the sacred art of gua sha, a practice that is not only powerful and restorative but deeply aligned with your divine feminine energy. Gua sha is all about reconnecting with your body, awakening your inner radiance and honouring yourself like the goddess you are.

Think of this guide as your sacred companion, here to help you unlock the magic of gua sha. Whether you're just beginning your journey or refining your technique, this is your time to take a moment to slow down, tune in and reclaim your personal ritual of self-care and empowerment.

You might wonder, "Isn't this easier to learn from a video?" While visual guides are helpful, they don't always teach you the why or the energy behind each movement, the deeper purpose of every stroke, or how this ritual helps you shift stagnant energy, move stress out of your body and awaken your true glow. This guide is designed to be more than instructions; it's a source of wisdom that you can return to again and again, helping you build confidence, trust your intuition and make this practice uniquely yours.

My goal is for you to feel empowered, confident and deeply connected to this ritual. Every goddess is unique, and your practice should reflect that. Allow yourself to experiment, to feel into what your body needs and to embrace the techniques that resonate most with you.

Understanding Gua Sha Principles

Before you even pick up your gua sha tool, it's important to know how to spot areas that need attention. Gua sha practitioners look for signs of stagnation and inflammation, often found in the neck, back and other tension-prone areas. You don't need to be an expert to identify these spots yourself.

Before we get into the technique, let's talk about something fundamental: *sha*. What is it, and why does it matter? Understanding sha is the key to making gua *sha* truly effective, helping you work *with* your body rather than just gliding a tool over your skin.

What is Sha?

Sha refers to the redness that often appears during gua sha, caused by stagnation in blood flow or energy (*Qi*). This stagnation could be the result of tension, tightness or blockages under the skin. Think of it like a river. When debris clogs the flow, the water slows down or even gets stuck. Similarly, stagnant Qi and blood flow can lead to pain, fatigue and even illness.

How do I Identify Sha?

You can check for *sha* before starting gua sha to get a sense of where your body might need extra attention:

1. Press a spot on your skin with your fingertips and release.

2. If the pale area takes longer than usual to fade, stagnation is present.

Why Address Sha?

When blood and energy aren't flowing properly, your body is more prone to tightness, discomfort and a general lack of vitality. Gua sha helps to release this stagnation, improve circulation and restore balance.

Preparing for Gua Sha

I've learnt that not all gua sha tools are created equal!

I once made the mistake of buying a cheap one from Amazon, and it turned out to be a complete disappointment. It wasn't real jade, had tiny abrasions that weren't great for my skin, and it broke almost immediately. Definitely not ideal!

Before you dive into gua sha, it's really important to set yourself up for success. Investing in a quality tool that feels comfortable and is designed to work well with your skin is key. And don't forget a good oil or serum – proper lubrication is essential for a smooth and effective practice.

After a long and frustrating search for the perfect gua sha tool, I realised I wanted something a bit different. I wanted a genuine stone with calming properties, a "U" shape that fits perfectly under the jawline and even ridges to help stimulate hair growth along the hairline. When I couldn't find what I was after, I decided to create it myself, and that's how the Freedom Gua Sha Tool came to be.

Choosing the Right Tool

Here's what to consider when picking the perfect tool:

Material Matters

Natural stones like jade, rose quartz or green aventurine aren't just beautiful, they're also durable, smooth and cool to the touch. They provide the perfect glide for your skin while adding a sense of luxury to your routine. Synthetic or poorly made tools, on the other hand, can irritate your skin or even break after a few uses.

I've always been drawn to the beauty of green aventurine, the way it feels smooth to the touch and carries a sense of calm. That's why I chose this premium stone for my gua sha design. Known for its stress-relieving and healing properties, green aventurine is often referred to as the stone of opportunity, helping to restore emotional balance and promote relaxation. It's the perfect companion for a gua sha ritual that's all about luxury, self-care and serenity.

Shape and Versatility

A great gua sha tool should fit comfortably in your hand and include various edges designed to contour your face and body. Curved edges are perfect for sculpting the jawline, while flat edges work beautifully for the forehead and cheeks.

My unique U-shaped gua sha tool is thoughtfully designed to lift and sculpt your jawline effortlessly. It also features ridges for deeper stimulation, making it ideal for areas such as the scalp or the back of your neck. Whether you're a beginner or an experienced practitioner, its ergonomic shape ensures a comfortable, precise glide every time.

Weight and Feel

A well-designed gua sha tool should feel balanced in your hand, neither too heavy nor too light. The right weight allows you to apply pressure comfortably without straining your wrist or fingers.

One of the most common frustrations I hear from friends and clients who've bought cheaper, lightweight gua shas is how easily they break. I've been there too! That's why I created the Freedom Gua Sha Tool with the perfect weight – solid enough to provide control and the right amount of pressure, while still feeling secure and effortless to use. A slightly heavier tool not only makes the technique easier but is also far more durable.

The U-shaped design and ideal weight of the Freedom Gua Sha Tool have made it a firm favourite. If you'd like to experience it for yourself, you can find it exclusively at www.shanti3.com.

Choosing the Right Oil

Never skip the oil! A good lubricant is essential for a smooth, effective gua sha practice, preventing unnecessary pulling or irritation. If you're uncomfortable with using oil, please use a moisturiser instead. The right oil not only helps your tool glide effortlessly but also nourishes your skin, leaving you with that post-gua sha glow.

Here's how to choose the best oil for your skin:

Texture and Viscosity

Look for oils that provide the right amount of slip, not too thick, not too watery. This ensures your tool glides effortlessly without clogging your pores or leaving a greasy residue.

Skin Type Compatibility

Oily or acne-prone skin? Go for lightweight, non-comedogenic oils like jojoba or argan, which won't block pores. Dry or mature skin? Richer oils like argan or sea buckthorn deliver deep hydration while soothing dry patches.

Ingredients to Avoid

Steer clear of synthetic fragrances, alcohol or harsh additives that can disrupt your skin's natural balance and counteract the benefits of gua sha. I created the SHANTI[3] Freedom Facial Oil specifically for gua sha, making it lightweight yet deeply hydrating, with a blend of botanical carrier oils that nourish the skin without clogging pores. Free from synthetic additives, it's gentle, effective and suitable for all skin types.

Lymphatic Drainage Massage

Before diving into your gua sha session, it's essential to prepare your body with a lymphatic drainage massage. This step might seem skippable, but trust me – it's the foundation of an effective gua sha routine. Think of it as clearing the path for your skin and body to reap the benefits of gua sha fully.

Why Lymphatic Drainage Is Important

The lymphatic system is like your body's natural detox network, quietly working to remove waste, toxins and excess fluid. However, stress, lack of movement or even general lifestyle habits can cause blockages, leading to puffiness, discomfort and even compromised immunity.

By stimulating the lymphatic system before gua sha, you create a clear, flowing pathway for stagnant fluid to drain away. This boosts your circulation, reduces swelling and enhances the sculpting and revitalising effects of gua sha. Without this step, the results of gua sha can be limited, as blocked pathways prevent proper drainage and circulation.

Why Preparation Is Non-Negotiable

You might be wondering, "Do I really need to do all this before gua sha?"

The answer is a resounding "yes".

Without first activating your lymph nodes and clearing blockages, gua sha can't deliver its full potential. Stagnant fluid will simply sit in place, leaving you with underwhelming results.

Think of it like unclogging a drain before running water. If you skip this crucial preparation step, everything backs up and nothing flows.

But with just a few minutes of lymphatic massage, you're setting the stage for gua sha magic to happen.

Lymphatic Drainage Leads to Immediate Gua Sha Results: A Story

It only takes a couple of minutes to properly open your lymph nodes, and the benefits of gua sha can start showing up after just one session. Don't believe me? Let me share a moment from my first two-day exhibition at a venue with over 20,000 attendees.

A mother and daughter approached my gua sha stand, looking curious but undeniably sceptical. The daughter, in her twenties, picked up the gua sha tool and asked, "What's this?" I introduced myself, the tool and my Freedom Facial Oil, sharing how gua sha can sculpt, lift and rejuvenate the skin. The daughter was intrigued enough to give it a try. Her mum, though, wasn't buying it – literally and figuratively. She rolled her eyes, saying, "You don't need that," clearly unimpressed by her daughter's love of beauty expos. It was one of those relatable moments that made us all laugh because, let's be honest, expos can be tough on the wallet!

I turned to the mum and said, "Alright, let's put it to the test. I'll work on just one side of her face, and you can decide if you see a difference." Challenge accepted. The daughter held up a mirror as I began.

We started with lymphatic drainage prep, which she admitted she'd never heard of. This step is essential; it's like clearing a blocked road before traffic can flow smoothly. By preparing her lymphatic system, I ensured that any excess fluid or stagnation in her face would drain away, leaving room for gua sha's lifting and sculpting magic to work. Then, I moved on to sculpting her jawline, lifting her cheekbones and raising her brow using precise, unidirectional strokes with the gua sha tool.

In just a few minutes, she gasped, "Oh wow!" Her mum, who had been glued to her phone, looked up, blinked and exclaimed, "Wait a second… one side of your face is different! Your jawline is sharper, your cheekbones are higher and your eyebrow looks lifted!" She couldn't believe the visible transformation. The daughter was equally stunned, staring at the mirror in awe. What had started as curiosity turned into a moment of conversion for both of them.

Long story short, they left with gua sha tools and facial oils in hand, completely convinced by the power of the demonstration. Moments like these are why I'm so passionate about gua sha, not as a fleeting beauty trend but as a lifestyle that combines traditional wisdom with modern wellness. When you understand the foundational techniques, gua sha becomes more than a skincare practice; it becomes a holistic ritual for healing, self-care and beauty.

How to Perform a Lymphatic Drainage Massage

Here's a simple, step-by-step guide to stimulate the lymph nodes and channels across your face and body. Take your time with each step. Remember that moderate pressure is key. Follow in chronological order for best results.

No.	Area	How	Why
1	Armpit Hollows	Use your thumbs to massage the hollows of your armpits in gentle, clockwise and anticlockwise circles. Perform this 20 times on each side.	These are major drainage points for lymphatic fluid in the upper body. Stimulating them helps clear blockages that can otherwise lead to stagnant fluid in your face and chest. It's normal to feel mild tenderness here, as soreness can indicate blockages.
2	Collarbone Area	Place your thumbs beneath your collarbones and massage in small clockwise and anticlockwise circles. Repeat 20 times on each side.	The collarbone area is another major drainage point. Activating these nodes helps lymph fluid flow from the face and neck into the chest for elimination.

No.	Area	How	Why
3	Under the Ear Lobes	Place your thumbs just below your earlobes and massage in clockwise and anticlockwise circles 20 times per side.	The lymph nodes near the ears are directly connected to fluid buildup in the face, especially the jawline and cheeks. Activating them helps reduce puffiness and tension in these areas.
4	Sides of the Mouth	Focus on the corners of your mouth. Use your thumbs to perform gentle, clockwise and anticlockwise circular motions for 20 repetitions.	This area connects to lymphatic channels that drain fluid from the mid-face and mouth region. Massaging here supports better circulation and detoxification.
5	Nostrils	Place your thumbs on either side of your nose and massage in clockwise and anticlockwise circles for 20 repetitions.	Stagnation around the nostrils is a common cause of puffiness and congestion in the under-eye area. Clearing these nodes can also promote sinus relief.

No.	Area	How	Why
6	Outer Corners of the Eyes	Gently massage the outer corners of your eyes in small, clockwise and anticlockwise circles 20 times per side.	This delicate area is prone to fluid build-up, often leading to puffiness and dark circles. Stimulating lymphatic flow in this area can visibly brighten and refresh the eyes.
7	Centre of the Forehead	Using your thumb, massage the middle of your forehead in clockwise and anticlockwise circles for 20 repetitions.	This step helps relax tension and stimulates the lymphatic channels that drain fluid from the forehead and brow area. It's also incredibly calming!

Let's do this together! Scan the QR code in the conclusion to follow along with my video tutorial.

Let's summarise the foundations for good gua sha technique so you can start experiencing these results for yourself.

Mastering the Gua Sha Technique

Gua sha is about understanding how energy flows, improving circulation and how to stimulate lymphatic drainage for maximum benefit. Here's a step-by-step guide to mastering the technique:

Start by identifying the areas you want to focus on. These are usually spots where you feel tension, puffiness or stagnation, like your jawline, cheeks or forehead. By targeting these zones, you're addressing the areas that need the most attention.

Next, prep your skin with a few drops of the Freedom Facial Oil. The oil is essential to ensure your gua sha tool glides smoothly and comfortably, without tugging or pulling. It will also nourish your skin, leaving it feeling hydrated and glowing.

Always use a facial oil or thick moisturiser so the tool glides easily over your skin. You should never feel pulling or discomfort.

When it comes to positioning the tool, hold it at a low angle, almost flat against your skin. This helps spread the pressure evenly and ensures a comfortable experience while still stimulating circulation.

Now, the most important part: the strokes.

You want to glide the tool in a long, steady motion (about 4 to 6 inches), repeating each stroke 10 times in a single direction. This consistency helps with lymphatic drainage, boosts blood circulation and helps reduce puffiness. Don't worry if you notice some redness; it's a good sign that the circulation is improving and not a sign of irritation.

Lastly, follow the "Above, Through, Below" rule. Start just above the area you're focusing on, gently stroke through it and finish just below. This ensures that you're moving fluid and energy in the right direction for the best results.

With a bit of practice, you'll find that gua sha becomes a truly restorative ritual, helping you relax, release tension and leave your skin glowing.

Are you ready to give it a try? Without further ado, let's explore the 10 steps for gua sha practice that I recommend incorporating into your daily ritual. These steps target the most commonly requested areas for gua sha, including the jawline and under-eye area – perfect for beginners!

10 Steps for Gua Sha Success

Ready to transform your skincare routine and experience the benefits of gua sha? Follow these 10 simple steps to sculpt, lift and rejuvenate your face and body while embracing a moment of relaxation.

For all steps below, apart from the eye area, use a medium pressure. For the eye area, use gentle pressure with the gua sha tool.

Let's do this together! Scan the QR code in the conclusion to follow along with my video tutorial.

Step 1: Prep Your Skin

Warm 4 to 5 drops of facial oil between the palms of your hands.

Gently massage the oil into your face and neck.

This step creates a smooth surface for the gua sha tool, preventing friction and making the massage feel comfortable and soothing.

Step 2: Define Your Jawline

Place the "U" shape part of the tool at your chin.

Hold the skin gently with your other hand and sweep the tool along your jawline toward the bottom of your ear.

Repeat 15 times on each side.

This helps reduce puffiness and tension in the jaw area, resulting in a more defined and sculpted jawline.

Step 3: Help Drain Puffiness Downwards

Starting at the chin, sweep the tool up along the jaw and around the ear.

Then glide the tool straight down the side of your neck to your shoulder.

Repeat 15 times per side.

This step directs lymphatic fluid toward your body's natural drainage points, helping reduce swelling and clear out toxins.

Step 4: Lift Your Cheekbones

Smile slightly to find your cheekbones.

Place one tip of the tool next to your nostril and the other at the corner of your mouth.

Sweep up across the cheekbone and out toward the top of your ear.

Repeat 15 times on each side.

This lifts and shapes your cheekbones, improving circulation.

Step 5: Drain Puffiness from Cheeks

Do the same sweep as Step 4, but extend the glide around the back of the ear, down the side of your neck, to your shoulder.

Repeat 15 times per side.

Adding the downward sweep helps clear built-up fluids, making your face look more contoured and refreshed.

Step 6: Refresh the Eye Area

Using the pointed tip of the tool, gently circle the outer corner of your eye 10 times.

Then glide the tool in an oval: from the outer brow to the inner corner, under the eye, and back to the starting point.

Gently circle the outer corner of the eye 10 times.

Repeat 10 times per eye.

This reduces puffiness, dark circles, and eye strain, leaving your eyes looking brighter and less tired.

Step 7: Relieve Sinus Pressure

With the pointed tip, circle the inner corner of your eye (near the nose) 10 times.

Sweep the tool from the side of your nose downward toward your nostrils.

Repeat 10 times per side.

These motions help clear sinus congestion and improve breathing. If your nose runs a bit afterwards, that's normal!

Step 8: Smooth Your Forehead

Using the long, curved edge, start at the centre of your forehead and sweep straight up toward your hairline.

Work section by section across the forehead.

Repeat 15 times per area.

This smooths out fine lines, relaxes tension (especially between the brows), and encourages collagen production.

Step 9: Release Neck Tension

Focus on the back of your neck.

Starting at the hairline, glide the tool downward to the base of your neck.

Repeat 10 times in the centre and on each side.

This relieves stiffness in the neck and shoulders, promoting better circulation and relaxation.

Step 10: Stimulate Your Scalp

Use the ridged edge of the tool to gently scrape along your hairline, moving back toward the crown of your head.

Work in sections around your whole scalp.

This boosts blood flow to the scalp, encouraging healthy hair growth and easing scalp tension.

Final Reminder

Take your time and enjoy the process! Gua sha isn't just about the results; it's also a calming ritual to help you slow down, relax and care for yourself.

By weaving gua sha into your daily routine, you'll not only sculpt and illuminate your skin but also awaken a profound sense of peace and self-love. Gua sha is a sacred act of self-honouring, a tool to release what no longer serves you and restore balance, not just to your skin but to your mind, heart and soul. When practised with intention, it transforms more than just your appearance. It shifts how you feel, how you carry yourself, and how you step into your power every single day.

To deepen your practice, explore our website and social media, where you'll find videos, tips and expert guidance to help you elevate your gua sha journey. (www.shanti3.com)

Let's dive into a few commonly asked questions to ensure you're equipped with all the knowledge you need for gua sha success.

Common Gua Sha FAQs

Should I Keep My Gua Sha Tool Cold in the Fridge?

No, it's not necessary to refrigerate your gua sha tool. In fact, using a cold tool goes against the principles of TCM, which emphasise the benefits of warmth and heat.

The friction created between the gua sha tool and your skin naturally generates heat. This warmth improves blood circulation and promotes lymphatic drainage, essential for reducing puffiness and enhancing skin health.

While many believe that a cold gua sha tool helps with puffiness, this is better achieved through the tool's massage technique, not its temperature. In summary, use your gua sha tool at room temperature for optimal benefits.

How Do I Clean My Gua Sha Tool?

Cleaning your gua sha tool is essential for hygiene and preventing bacteria from transferring to your skin. Here's how to clean your gua sha tool, step-by-step:

1. After use, wipe off any remaining facial oil from the tool using a soft, clean cloth or kitchen towel.

2. Wash the tool in warm, soapy water (not boiling). Use a gentle soap to avoid damaging the material.

3. Allow the tool to air-dry completely by placing it on a clean kitchen towel. Avoid storing it while damp.

Don't forget to wash your hands thoroughly before using your gua sha tool. The tool needs to be cleaned after every use to maintain cleanliness and prevent breakouts or irritation.

Is It Better to Use Gua Sha in the Morning or Evening?

This depends on your schedule and personal preference, as both morning and evening sessions offer unique benefits.

For morning benefits, start your day with a 5 to 10 minute gua sha ritual to relieve tension in your jaw, reduce puffiness and energise your skin. A morning ritual also provides a moment of mindfulness, helping you stay calm as you tackle a busy day.

For evening benefits, a relaxing gua sha session at the end of the day can help release tension accumulated throughout the day, ease facial tightness and promote better sleep.

For maximum results, you can use gua sha just after you shower. When your skin is damp and warm, pores are open, allowing for greater efficacy of oil absorption and more effective gua sha practice.

Is Gua Sha Safe?

Yes, gua sha is a safe technique with a long history of use in TCM. However, there are certain situations where caution or professional advice is required.

If you are under 16 or over 70 years old, consult a medical practitioner before use. If approved, it's best to have someone else perform the technique for you.

Avoid gua sha if you're feeling unwell, taking certain medications or have undergone surgery within the past year. Always consult your doctor in such cases.

Do not use gua sha on areas with:

- Broken skin, moles, cuts or bruises
- Thread veins or varicose veins
- Any existing skin condition causing discomfort or irritation

It's also important to note that gua sha should never be painful. If you experience significant discomfort, stop immediately and review your technique.

How Often Should I Practice Gua Sha?

Gua sha can be safely practised daily for 5 to 10 minutes, making it a manageable and effective addition to your skincare routine.

The best time to perform gua sha is right after a warm shower. The heat opens your pores, allowing your skin to absorb facial oil more effectively. This enhances the benefits of the gua sha massage, including improved hydration and faster skin repair.

Regular, consistent use helps promote glowing skin, reduces stress and enhances overall wellbeing by incorporating mindfulness into your daily routine.

By making this a daily ritual, you'll start to notice less tension, a deeper sense of calm and long-term improvements in your skin's texture.

For more exclusive gua sha videos, just scan the QR code in the conclusion, or join us on Instagram at https://www.instagram.com/shanti3official for fresh tips and inspiration!

Chapter 6

RELIEF FROM COMMON MENOPAUSAL SYMPTOMS

Menopause can feel like an emotional rollercoaster, leaving you wondering where your sense of balance and vitality has gone. Hot flushes, bloating and sudden discomfort can make you feel disconnected from your own body, as if a storm is brewing within.

But what if I told you there's a powerful, transformative tool that can help you navigate these changes with ease, while reconnecting to your inner strength and wisdom? The answer lies in gua sha. Gua sha technique isn't about complicated solutions or expensive treatments. Rather, it's about coming back home to your body, nurturing it with intention and reclaiming the power to thrive through this transition.

Now, let's be clear: Gua sha isn't a magic cure. Just like brushing your teeth or exercising regularly, it's a consistent practice that invites real change over time. But when you approach gua sha with presence and care, treating it as a sacred ritual, you create space for deep transformation. By dedicating time to this ancient ritual, you can not only ease menopausal symptoms like hot flushes and bloating but also shift your mindset to one of empowerment and self-love.

Gua sha works to release tension, sculpt your features and restore a deep sense of calm. This practice goes beyond the surface; it's about reclaiming your body and embracing your inner strength. When you show up for yourself in this way, you're stepping into your divine feminine energy – radiant, grounded and in control.

Gua Sha as Daily Maintenance, a Ritual of Self-Love

From a young age, we're taught the importance of brushing our teeth daily. Just two minutes, twice a day, protects us from future dental issues. Over a lifetime, we spend around 38.5 days brushing our teeth. Gua sha operates on the same principle as a small, consistent act of self-care that prevents bigger issues from arising.

Rather than scrambling for relief when symptoms strike, gua sha allows you to build a steady, nurturing ritual that supports your body and mind. With just a few minutes each day, you can release tension, reduce discomforts like hot flushes and bloating, and feel more at ease within your body. This mindful ritual transforms menopause from something to endure into something to embrace. It's a time of awakening, resilience and renewal.

Imagine gliding through this phase of life with grace and confidence, breaking free from the myth that menopause must be a struggle. You are a goddess, and you deserve to feel radiant and powerful at every stage of your journey. Gua sha is your secret weapon to help you reclaim that beauty, comfort and confidence, because you are truly worthy of it.

Gua Sha Moves to Relieve Hot Flushes

Hot flushes can hit you like a sudden wave of heat, leaving you sweaty, flushed and overwhelmed. They're unpredictable, exhausting and downright frustrating. But gua sha can help. These three simple moves are designed to release built-up heat in your body, providing fast and effective relief when you need it most. The best part? You can do them anytime, anywhere.

Step 1: Relieve Heat From Your Head

Start by focusing on the heat building at the top of your head, a common hotspot during hot flushes.

How to Do It

- Imagine a straight line extending directly upward from the top centre of your head. This spot is where you'll start the motion. Think of it as the source of heat radiating outward.

- Hold your gua sha tool firmly, using the tip of the "U" shaped end. This part is perfect for making precise, gliding motions on your head.

- Place the tip gently on the top, centre of your head. Apply moderate pressure, just enough to feel the tool working but without causing discomfort.

- Glide the tool downward in a single, sweeping motion from your head to the top of your ear. Keep the movement smooth and steady.

- Complete 8 to 10 strokes along this path, moving from your head to the top of one ear.

- After finishing the first section, return to the centre of your head. Adjust the angle of your strokes slightly and repeat the motion toward the level of the top of your ear.

- Work systematically around your head, covering all angles – front, back and sides – while always gliding the tool downward towards the level of the top of the ear.

- Each new direction should have at least 8 to 10 repetitions.

Continue the technique as long as necessary, repeating strokes until you feel the heat start to dissipate. The goal is to cover as much of the head as possible while gradually cooling down. This technique helps "pull" the heat away from your head and direct it downward, cooling your body. You'll feel an immediate sense of relief as the heat moves away from your crown.

Step 2: Cool Behind Your Ears

The area behind your ears is a powerful cooling point connected to the body's heat-regulating pathways. This move enhances the cooling effect from Step 1.

How to Do It

- Gently pull your ear out to the side with one hand.

- With your gua sha tool in the other hand, scrape downward behind your ear, starting from the top and moving toward the bottom.

- Repeat for a minimum of 10 strokes on each side.

This technique helps release heat and tension stored in the sensitive area behind your ears, further lowering your internal temperature.

Step 3: Target the Mid to Lower Back

Heat often accumulates in the mid and lower back during a hot flush. Addressing this area not only cools you down but also relieves tension.

How to Do It

- Locate the mid-back (just below your ribcage) and lower back (just above your hips).

- Using the long edge of your gua sha tool, glide it in a straight motion from the mid-back down toward the lower back.

- Repeat the motion for at least 8 to 10 strokes per area.

This step also works wonders for abdominal discomfort or tension, making it perfect for days when bloating and discomfort accompany hot flushes.

Real Life Relief

At a pop-up event, I met a lovely woman who was experiencing a hot flush. She was sweating, her curly hair was damp and the warmth radiating from her head was quite noticeable. She was a little unsure when I suggested trying gua sha, but she decided to give it a go.

I began with Step 1, gently gliding the gua sha tool from the top of her head towards her ears, repeating each stroke about 10 times. As I worked, I could see her body begin to relax. Her hot flush started to subside, and not only did she feel cooler, but she also felt a sense of calm. There was no need to move on to the next steps; she was already feeling so much better. She looked at me, surprised and relieved, and said, "I wish I'd known about this sooner!"

Her experience isn't unique. Gua sha has helped so many women feel better, and it can do the same for you, too.

Did you know that our emotions are often linked to specific parts of our body? When we're under stress or feeling overwhelmed, our body tends to hold onto those emotions, especially when it feels like the right time to deal with them hasn't come yet.

However, when we don't allow ourselves to fully process or release those emotions, they get stored physically in our bodies. Your body truly is a reflection of your mind. If you're experiencing digestive issues or feeling tightness in your chest, it could be a sign that these unprocessed emotions are waiting to be acknowledged and healed. A wonderful way to begin this healing process is through gua sha.

Gua Sha for Your Stomach

Bloating, let's be honest, is never comfortable. Whether it's caused by indigestion, hormonal changes, the stresses of menopause or even emotions that haven't been fully processed, we've all experienced it. And regardless of your age, it's always frustrating to feel bloated. For many women, this can become even more challenging during menopause.

The emotions connected to discomfort in the stomach, like indigestion, bloating or pain, can often come from feelings of being unable to express your power, ongoing stress, negative self-talk or even frustration and anxiety. If this resonates with you, please know that you're not alone. Many women struggle with digestive discomfort, especially during this stage of life. If you're looking for some relief, gua sha can be a gentle and soothing way to ease that bloating. A simple stomach massage using this technique can support your digestion, reduce bloating and help you feel more comfortable and at ease again.

How to Do It

You'll need a gua sha tool and a few drops of oil. You can do this while standing or lying on your back, whichever position feels more comfortable for you. Avoid sitting as it restricts movement.

To make this easier, imagine your stomach is divided into three sections:

Upper: From your ribs down to your belly button.

Naval: Slightly above and below the belly button.

Lower: From below the belly button to just above the pelvic bone.

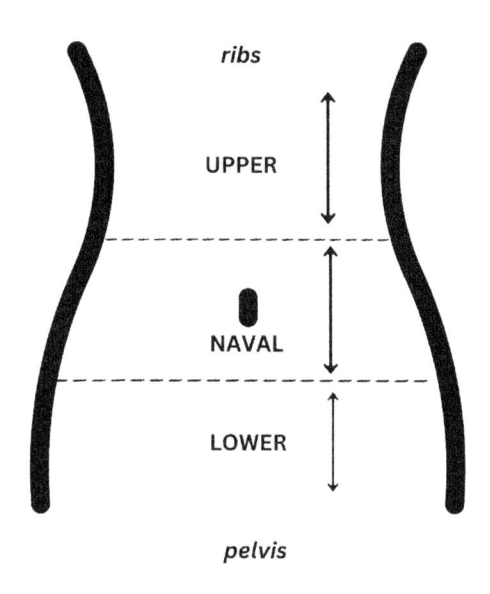

```
         ribs
          ↑
        UPPER
          ↓
    - - - - - - - -
          ↑
     ▮  NAVAL
          ↓
    - - - - - - - -
          ↑
        LOWER
          ↓
         pelvis
```

Step 1: Apply Oil to Your Stomach

- Start by applying a few drops of oil to your stomach so the gua sha tool glides smoothly.

This prevents friction, making the massage more comfortable and effective.

Step 2: Massage the Upper Stomach

- Place your non-dominant (supporting) hand just under your ribcage.

- Using the long edge of the gua sha tool in your other hand, gently stroke downward toward your belly button, in a vertical motion, moving downward.

- Repeat this 10 times with moderate pressure.

This helps release tension in the upper stomach and encourages trapped gas or air to move downward, giving you relief.

Step 3: Massage Around the Belly Button

- Place your supporting hand above the belly button.

- Use the gua sha tool to stroke downwards over the belly button. Again, use a vertical motion, moving downward.

- Repeat 10 times with moderate pressure.

The area around the belly button can hold a lot of bloating, so this motion helps move things along.

Step 4: Massage the Lower Stomach

- Place your supporting hand below the belly button.

- With the gua sha tool, stroke vertically and downward toward your pelvic bone.

- Repeat 10 times with moderate pressure.

This helps release tension and supports natural digestion and elimination.

Step 5: Repeat on the Sides of Your Stomach

- Repeat Steps 2, 3, and 4 on the left and right sides of your abdomen.

- If you feel any discomfort, slow down and move gently until the area starts to ease.

This helps relieve tension across the entire stomach and supports overall gut health.

Step 6: Circular Massage Around the Belly Button

- Use the long edge of the gua sha tool to make gentle clockwise circles around your belly button.

- Repeat 10 times with moderate pressure.

Moving clockwise follows the natural path of your intestines, helping to get digestion moving and reduce bloating.

Step 7: Glide from the Waist to the Belly Button

- Place the gua sha tool at the side of your waist.

- Glide it horizontally toward your belly button, moving inward.

- Repeat 10 times on each side with moderate pressure.

This encourages digestion and helps release trapped wind, giving you a flatter, more comfortable stomach.

Step 8: Scrape Up and Down Along the Waist

- Place the gua sha tool at the sides of your waist and scrape upward and downward, moving vertically.

- Repeat 10 times on each side with moderate pressure.

This relieves tension in the lower back, improves circulation, and helps sculpt the waistline.

When Should You Do This?

Doing this in the morning is perfect for kickstarting your digestion and encouraging bowel movements, helping you feel lighter and more comfortable as you start your day.

An evening routine, on the other hand, is ideal for easing tension, relaxing your body and winding down for a restful night's sleep.

My personal recommendation is to try this stomach-debloating technique first thing in the morning. It's a great way to stimulate digestion, reduce bloating and set yourself up for a day of feeling your best.

Reclaiming Your Radiance: A Gua Sha Story

Struggling to find the perfect outfit for a party? We've all been there: standing in front of the wardrobe, pulling out outfit after outfit, searching for something that feels comfortable yet radiates confidence. The frustration of thinking, "I have nothing to wear!" is all too familiar.

That's exactly where I found myself during a recent staycation in the UK. My sister and I were getting ready for dinner, and everyone was dressing to impress. I had two choices: a stunning black off-the-shoulder dress that always made me feel empowered, or a "safe" option – trousers, a nice top and a jumper. Naturally, my heart longed for the black dress.

But as I slipped it on, I caught sight of my reflection and froze.

All I could focus on was my bloated stomach. You know the feeling. After indulging in a few days of delicious food, your body feels heavy and nothing fits quite right. The dress, which had once made me feel powerful and feminine, now felt restrictive and unforgiving. Self-doubt crept in. Should I cover up? Should I hide myself away?

I was on the verge of swapping to the "safe" outfit when I remembered something: I already have the power to transform how I feel in my body. My Freedom Gua Sha Tool and Freedom Facial Oil were packed in my bag. Why not give myself the same care and love I always encourage others to give to themselves?

I lay down, applied the oil to my stomach and began a gentle lymphatic drainage massage with my gua sha. The shift was incredible. Within minutes, I could feel my body responding to the motions. The tightness eased, the discomfort lifted and I could sense the stagnant energy and fluid beginning to move. But it wasn't just a physical release, it was an energetic one too. I felt lighter, more at ease and deeply connected to my body again.

After finishing, I slipped back into the black dress and looked in the mirror. This time, I smiled. The bloating had visibly reduced, my stomach felt firmer and more toned, and, most importantly, I felt like myself again. Even my sister noticed, saying, "Wow! What a difference!"

That dress, which had felt like my enemy just moments before, now became a symbol of my power. I paired it with my heels and stepped out for dinner, not just looking confident, but feeling it, because I had chosen to honour my body rather than criticise it.

Why It's Worth Trying

This practice isn't just about easing bloating. It supports your digestion, nurtures gut health and restores internal balance. This is especially important during menopause, when everything can feel a little out of sync. Gua sha is a gentle, effective way to reconnect with your body, ease discomfort and anchor yourself in your feminine strength.

So, whether you're dealing with bloating after a big meal, monthly cramps or the hormonal shifts of menopause, this ancient ritual is worth embracing. It's a small yet powerful act of self-respect: a way to honour your body, awaken your vitality and move through life with more ease, grace and confidence.

Gua sha is a tool for self-reclamation, and not just about sculpted skin or temporary relief. It reminds you that you are in control of how you feel in your body. Whether you're preparing for a special event or simply seeking to reconnect on a quiet evening, it's about showing up for yourself with love, presence and intention.

At the end of the day, confidence isn't just about the outfit. It's about the woman wearing it and the power she chooses to embody.

Chest Scraping with Gua Sha

As women, we tend to store emotions and stress in our chest area. When we are triggered, any residual, unprocessed emotions that our mind holds form physical tension around the chest area. Gua sha for your chest can help alleviate anxiety and stress during menopause. This is why the Goddess Meditation Ritual is essential for tapping into your calm, so that you can live each day in your divine goddess energy.

If you continuously feel anxious or stressed, the tension builds and can cause pain, inflammation and worry.

Fear not, this is one of the most underrated gua sha techniques, but my favourite. A goddess knows that her mindset is the most important to her overall wellbeing.

If you want to embody your divine feminine energy every day, this gua sha technique is for you. It's the ultimate life hack to alleviate anxiety in a matter of minutes, and even if you're not feeling anxious, worried or stressed, this gua sha technique acts as a maintenance ritual.

Chest scraping has many benefits; it can calm you down, stop those racing thoughts and help you sleep. It feels wonderful, too, as it relieves pressure from wearing a bra! If you're feeling congested in your chest from a cough or build-up of phlegm, this technique can even break down mucus stored in your chest area.

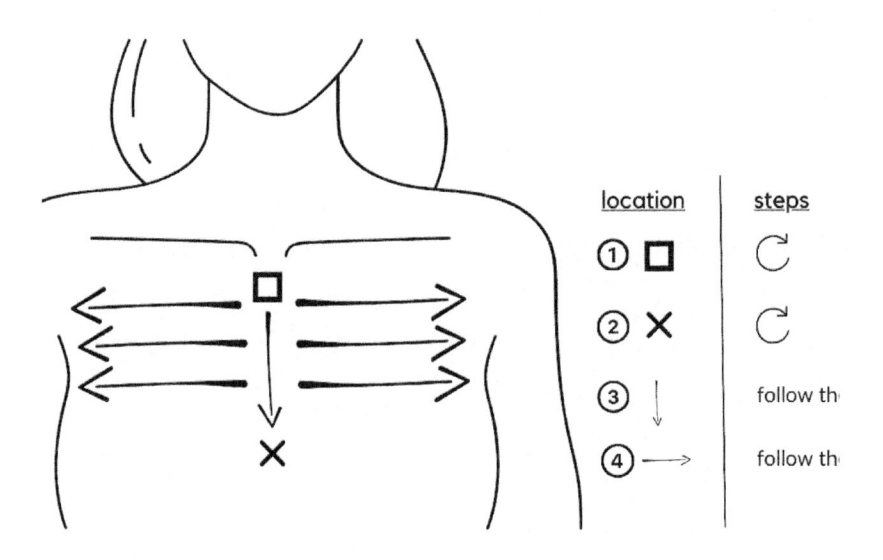

location	steps
① □	C
② ✕	C
③ ↓	follow th
④ →	follow th

150 | GLOW THROUGH THE CHANGE

How to Do It

Begin with your Lymphatic Drainage massage, with a particular focus on massaging the area under your armpits to open up the lymph nodes. As usual, take a couple of drops of oil and make sure the chest area is properly lubricated.

Repeat steps 1 to 4 at least 20 times.

Step 1: Start at the centre of your chest

- Start at the '☐', or the centre where your collarbones meet.

- Use your gua sha tool to massage this acupressure point in a clockwise direction.

You can work here longer if you feel emotions pouring out of you. Let that tension go!

Step 2: Massage the acupressure point between your breasts

- Start at the "X" or the acupressure point between your breasts.

- Use your gua sha tool to massage this acupressure point in a clockwise direction.

It may feel tender to the touch.

Step 3: Move from the centre of your chest downwards between your breasts

- Start at the '☐' or the centre where your collarbones meet.

- Follow the direction of the arrow vertically down ending at the 'X'.

It's completely normal if redness starts to appear.

Step 4: Move from the centre of your chest outwards to the sides

- Start at the centre of your chest.

- Glide your gua sha horizontally across your chest towards your underarm.

- Repeat on each side.

Make sure to continue the gua sha movement finishing at the armpit area so that the lymphatic fluid can drain.

Gua Sha for the Heart Space

As women, we are vessels of energy, wisdom, and intuition. We carry so much within us – our emotions, our worries, our unspoken thoughts – and often, these find a home in our bodies, particularly in our chest. This is the sacred space of the heart, where love, grief, joy and burdens all reside. During menopause, when emotions can feel heightened and the body is undergoing so many changes, this stored tension can manifest as anxiety, stress or even physical discomfort.

It's as if the weight of lifetimes, of nurturing, of giving, of holding space for others, has settled within you, making it harder to breathe deeply, to feel free and to reconnect with the vibrant, empowered woman you truly are. Gua sha for the chest allows you to release some of that weight, soothing both body and mind. It's an incredibly powerful technique, yet one of the most underrated. I truly believe it's something every woman should experience, not just during moments of heightened stress or anxiety, but as a daily act of self-care – a sacred moment to honour your heart centre, where so much emotional truth is held.

Many women move through menopause without taking back the reins. They brace themselves for symptoms, feeling as though they have no choice but to endure. But not you. You're choosing differently. You are reclaiming your inner power. You honour your sacred body, listening to its whispers and responding with care. You choose to meet yourself daily with compassion and intention, living from a place of presence and feminine strength.

In just a few minutes, it can bring an immediate sense of relief, grounding you in the present moment, like the stillness of the ocean after a storm – calm, expansive and at peace. Even if you don't feel particularly stressed or anxious, it works as a beautiful maintenance ritual, keeping emotions moving rather than letting them settle into tightness and tension. Just as a river remains pure by flowing freely, our emotions must do the same to stay in harmony.

Beyond its emotional benefits, chest scraping with gua sha can help with a range of physical discomforts, too. It eases that feeling of constriction from wearing a bra all day, relieves built-up pressure in the chest, and even helps to break down congestion if you're suffering from a cough or a build-up of mucus. But perhaps most importantly, it encourages emotional release, a softening of the armour we unknowingly carry. If you've been feeling weighed down, as though you're carrying a burden that no one else can see, this practice can offer a deep sense of lightness.

It helps to shift emotions that often lodge themselves in the chest – feelings of overwhelm, exhaustion, unspoken sorrow or the ache of giving too much without receiving enough in return. If you've been struggling to express yourself, feeling like life is spinning out of control, or noticing heightened sensitivity to stress, this practice may become your anchor, a ritual that brings you back home to yourself.

Menopause is more than just a physical transition; it is an initiation, a rebirth into a new phase of feminine power. In the midst of daily responsibilities, it's easy to move through life without stopping to process what you're feeling. But a goddess does not suppress her emotions. Instead, she honours them, she listens and she allows them to flow.

It helps to think of it in terms of one of the most fundamental laws of nature: Newton's Third Law. For every action, there is an equal and opposite reaction. If you are constantly giving – pouring energy into your tasks, your family, your work, your responsibilities – without allowing yourself the space to receive, to rest and to reflect, your body will eventually push back. You cannot pour from an empty chalice.

Things that may have once felt manageable, like stress at work or tension at home, may suddenly feel overwhelming. Menopause heightens emotional responses, making it even more important to create moments where you can reconnect with yourself, where you can listen to the whispers of your body before they become shouts.

So, how do you process your emotions during menopause? How do you create that space for yourself?

Gua sha is one of the simplest, most effective ways to carry out a goddess ritual. With each stroke, you are giving yourself permission to pause, to breathe, to release. It is a ritual of self-reverence, a moment where you place yourself at the altar of your own wellbeing. As you move the tool across your chest, you may notice areas of redness appear, like a map revealing where your body has been holding onto tension, where energy has been waiting to be freed. And as the tightness dissolves, so too may the racing thoughts, the restlessness, the unease.

If, even after gua sha, you find emotions still sitting heavily within you, it may help to bring in other practices of self-expression. Journaling can be a portal to your soul, a way to unravel the knots within. Writing down your thoughts, first thing in the morning or just before bed, can offer clarity, helping you untangle emotions that otherwise feel overwhelming.

Speaking with a trusted friend, a healer or a loved one can also be transformative. When we voice our feelings, we free them. We reclaim our agency. Because empowered women do not suffer in silence. They reach out. They allow themselves to be supported, knowing that there is strength in vulnerability.

If you've ever felt stuck, like something deep inside is holding you back, you're not alone. ThetaHealing® offers a gentle yet powerful way to uncover and release the emotional blocks that keep you from moving forward. If you're ready to shift, heal and reconnect with yourself, I'd be honoured to support you. Learn more at www.shanti3.com.

These practices – gua sha, journaling, talking – are not just acts of self-care. They are acts of self-honouring.

Think of how you would care for a child going through a big life transition: with patience, kindness and compassion. You, too, deserve that same devotion. Menopause is an opportunity to treat yourself with that same tenderness, to honour the changes you are going through, rather than resist them.

Chapter 7
ENHANCING GUA SHA WITH THE RIGHT FACIAL OIL

Are you feeling excited and ready to embrace the gua sha technique? That's fantastic! You're learning a new skill and stepping into a sacred ritual of self-love, a moment where you honour your goddess energy. As you embark on this transformative journey, there's one final piece of wisdom you need: choosing the right facial oil to elevate your practice.

You can't just pick up any old bottle off the shelf. Your skin is a temple and it deserves intention, care and nourishment. During menopause, when hydration becomes unpredictable and your skin's needs shift like the tides, the right oil isn't just a luxury; it's an essential act of devotion to yourself.

Let me introduce a dear friend of mine, Siobhan. Siobhan is a mother to two grown-up beautiful girls, Clara and Sienna, a close family friend and one of my best friends. For years, she curated the most meticulous skincare ritual I've ever seen – luxurious products, high-end facials and a bathroom shelf lined with the finest elixirs. But even the most devoted goddess can feel unbalanced when menopause arrives, shifting the skin, the body and the spirit in unexpected ways.

Friday night. Siobhan's kitchen.

A bottle of wine open on the counter, two glasses half full, the scent of something rich and slow-cooked still hanging in the air. Siobhan leans back on her chair, sitting adjacent to me on a gorgeous wooden dining table, swirling her drink, that familiar crease forming between her brows.

"I don't know what's happening to my skin," she sighs, pressing her fingertips over her cheeks. "It's dry, tight…itchy. No matter what I use, nothing absorbs. It's like my skin's rejecting everything."

This, from the woman who has always had the most meticulous skincare routine I've ever known. She's spent years investing in the best of the best – Sisley, Shiseido, La Mer. The luxury brands with the hefty price tags, the ones promising hydration, radiance, eternal youth in a bottle.

But now? Menopause has other ideas.

"Even my facial oil isn't cutting it," she says, exasperated. "I used to swear by it, but now? My skin just drinks it up and still feels parched."

I take a slow sip of my wine, considering.

"I think you need to strip it all back," I say finally. "Just for a week. Use nothing but this." I pull a small glass pipette bottle from my bag. It's my own facial oil, a formula I've been perfecting, tweaking and testing on my own skin.

She raises an eyebrow but takes the bottle, rolling it between her fingers. "Seven days? Just this?"

"Seven days," I nod.

A week later, we're back in the same kitchen, another bottle of wine, another deep chat about life, work and now – skin.

"It's working," she says, running a hand over her cheek. "My skin actually feels hydrated again. Softer. But…," she holds the bottle up, inspecting the amber liquid. "The colour. Do you reckon you could make it a bit…less orange?"

She's right, the sea buckthorn oil gives it a rich golden hue. Not a dealbreaker, but a tweakable detail. Back to the drawing board I go, refining, adjusting and making sure the facial oil isn't just great for dry, menopausal skin, but also gentle enough for sensitive skin like mine.

But here's where it gets really interesting. As we start picking apart the ingredients in her high-end products, something becomes painfully obvious: a lot of them aren't actually worth the price.

Fancy branding, beautiful packaging, but when you strip all that away? The quality? Average.

So, she suggests we do a side-by-side test – her £200 facial oil versus my Freedom Facial Oil. She dabs a little of each onto the back of her hands, feeling the texture, the absorption, the finish. Then she looks up at me and grins.

"Yours is better."

And that, right there, is when we start asking the real questions.

What actually makes a good facial oil? What separates the ones that work from the ones that just look pretty on a bathroom shelf?

In menopause, there's no time for empty promises. Your skin is changing, and your skincare needs to keep up. It's not about what's trendy or expensive; it's about what delivers.

Why Does the Right Oil Matter?

When it comes to gua sha, the oil you choose is just as important as the tool itself. The right oil provides the perfect amount of slip, allowing the tool to glide effortlessly across your skin without tugging or pulling. Too little oil, and you risk dragging the skin, which can lead to irritation. Too much, and the tool slips too fast, making it harder to control, and far more likely to end up on the floor – not ideal!

The key is balance. You need to choose a facial oil that not only enhances your gua sha practice but also deeply nourishes and supports your menopausal skin. Hydration, elasticity and glow without the gimmicks.

So, as you begin your gua sha journey, ask yourself: Is your facial oil working for you? Or just sitting pretty on your shelf?

How Do You Fit Gua Sha Into Your Routine?

For my ladies who aren't too familiar with how to incorporate a facial oil in their skincare routine, I'm happy to let you know that using a facial oil is easy. The perfect time is right after your shower, when your skin is damp and your pores are open. Apply four to five drops of facial oil into clean palms, press gently into your face and start your gua sha ritual. Afterwards, follow up with your serum and cream, whether it's morning or evening. If it's a morning routine, simply add sunscreen and makeup on top.

Don't worry about wiping off the oil; it works beautifully under makeup, leaving your skin with a dewy, radiant glow. Trust me: Some of the best compliments I get are on days when I've practised gua sha and layered makeup over my facial oil.

But here's the tricky part: finding a facial oil that works for menopausal skin.

Hormonal shifts during menopause can wreak havoc on your complexion. The moisturiser you've relied on for over twenty years might suddenly feel useless, leaving you frustrated, confused and overwhelmed by the endless product choices. Maybe you've asked a friend for advice, only to try their expensive recommendation and find it's not the right fit. But your skin is uniquely yours. It deserves products tailored to its changing needs.

Navigating Skincare With Wisdom and Confidence

When it comes to skincare, menopausal skin has its own unique needs. It's often drier, more sensitive and prone to irritation or hormonal breakouts. With so many products on the market, it's easy to feel overwhelmed or swayed by marketing buzzwords like "clean", "natural", or "anti-ageing". However, understanding ingredients gives you the power to make informed, healthy choices for your skin.

Rather than chasing miracle products, this is the time to come home to your skin, to simplify, to nourish and to choose ingredients that work with your body, not against it. Let's explore how to do just that, with clarity and confidence.

For the full checklist, see Appendix 1 (Your Guide to Menopausal Skincare) at the back of the book.

Choose Ingredients That Truly Care for Your Skin

During menopause, your skin thrives when it's well-hydrated, protected and gently supported. Look for ingredients that offer genuine nourishment.

Moisture magnets. Plant-derived hyaluronic acid, glycerine and squalane replenish hydration and restore softness.

Botanical oils. Jojoba, argan, moringa and sea buckthorn provide deep nourishment, rich in antioxidants and essential fatty acids that support repair and regeneration.

Barrier-strengthening actives. These include shea butter, plant-based ceramides and essential fatty acids, which help your skin remain resilient and less reactive.

Antioxidants. Vitamin E, Coenzyme Q10 and green tea extract protect your skin from environmental damage and help slow visible signs of ageing.

And for those days when your skin feels flushed or reactive, soothing botanicals like chamomile, rosewater and passionflower bring comfort and calm.

These ingredients do more than moisturise. They support your skin's natural rhythm, helping it adapt, strengthen and glow.

Know What to Avoid

As your skin becomes more reactive during menopause, knowing what *not* to use is just as important. Fragrances, whether synthetic or naturally derived, are common irritants. Even natural compounds such as linalool and limonene can trigger redness and sensitivity.

It's also wise to steer clear of:

Harsh preservatives. Parabens and phenoxyethanol.

Drying alcohols. Ethanol or denatured alcohol.

Artificial colourants. These offer no benefit and may cause irritation.

Over-processed oils. These can be exchanged for cold-pressed, unrefined oils to retain nutrients and avoid potential skin stress.

Choosing simpler, purer formulations makes all the difference for skin that's adapting to hormonal changes.

Keep Your Routine Simple and Effective

> Look for the following:
>
> - **Short ingredient lists**
>   ideally under 10 to 12 ingredients
>
> - **Cold-pressed, unrefined oils**
>   for nutrient-rich nourishment
>
> - **Water-free balms or oils**
>   which tend to be richer and don't require synthetic preservatives

When it comes to skincare during this time, less is often more. A minimalist approach reduces the risk of irritation and helps you focus on what really works.

Gentle, well-formulated products can give your skin everything it needs, without unnecessary fillers or complexity.

Understand What You're Buying

Reading product labels might feel daunting at first, but with a little knowledge, it becomes second nature and incredibly empowering.

Keep these basics in mind:

- Ingredients are listed in order of concentration. If the hero ingredient is near the bottom, it's probably just there for marketing.

- Choose fragrance-free or unscented products to minimise the risk of irritation.

- If hormonal breakouts are a concern, opt for non-comedogenic oils like rosehip or hemp seed oil.

- Look for rich, creamy textures in moisturisers, and always choose non-foaming, pH-balanced cleansers to maintain your skin's natural barrier.

Understanding formulations helps you shop smart and care for your skin with confidence.

Introduce Products Slowly and Mindfully

Your skin is evolving, and it deserves patience. Introduce new products gradually. Patch test first by applying a small amount to your inner arm or jawline and waiting 24 hours to check for any reaction.

Then, observe how your skin responds over a few days. If it feels calm, hydrated and comfortable, it's likely a good fit.

Menopausal skin can be unpredictable at times, so this cautious approach helps you avoid setbacks and discover what truly works for you.

Create Rituals, Not Just Routines

Stick to your routine. Natural ingredients may work gradually, but they bring lasting benefits.

Also, incorporate calm. Stress affects your skin just as much as any product. Breathwork, music or a few moments of stillness can elevate your skincare into a true act of self-care.

Finally, consistency matters, but so does pleasure. Skincare doesn't have to be a chore. It can be grounding, soothing and even joyful. Whether it's massaging with a facial oil and your gua sha tool or simply applying moisturiser with care, these small moments can become sacred pauses in your day.

This is not about achieving perfection. It's about building a connection to your skin, your body and the woman you are becoming.

Janelle's Story

For months, she'd been battling stubborn, textured bumps on her skin. She was frustrated, confused and feeling like nothing was working. Every new product she tried seemed to make things worse.

One evening, as we sat down to chat about her skincare routine, a pattern started to emerge. The problem wasn't her skin; it was the combination of products she was using.

Like many of us, she'd been lured in by persuasive skincare sales reps, layering acids upon acids without fully understanding how they worked together. She thought she had combination skin – oily in the T-zone, dry on the cheeks – so she built a routine around that assumption. But when she stripped everything back and reset her skin, something surprising happened.

By introducing gentle, natural ingredients, like rosewater as a toner, she discovered the truth.

Her skin wasn't a combination. It was dry.

Just like our hormones, our skin can change over time. The key is to listen to it, read ingredient labels and notice how it reacts to products. If your skin starts feeling irritated, tight or out of balance, sometimes the best thing you can do is pause. Give your skin a break, return to basics, and gradually reintroduce products.

Because when you strip away the noise, the trends and the complicated routines, it becomes clear: Your skin will always tell you what it needs - you just have to pay attention.

Empowered Skincare Choices

Appendix 1 serves as your guide to navigating the complex world of skincare and making informed, healthy choices tailored to menopausal skin. By prioritising natural, fragrance-free ingredients and avoiding unnecessary irritants, you'll protect your skin's barrier, restore hydration and nurture its natural balance.

With knowledge comes empowerment, because you deserve skincare that works *for* you, not against you.

Take control of your routine, trust the process and give your skin the love, care and attention it needs to thrive during this transformative time.

Creating the Freedom Facial Oil

At the start of my gua sha journey, I faced a challenge: finding the *perfect* facial oil to complement my gua sha practice. My skin was in crisis. It had broken out into a rash, was painfully sensitive, extremely dry and allergic to even the smallest trace of fragrance. On top of that, I desperately wanted something that could breathe life into my dull, pale and lacklustre complexion.

I could have chosen a single carrier oil, such as jojoba, argan or rosehip, to use during gua sha. But I wanted to be smarter and more intentional with my skincare. By creating my own oil blend, I realised I could take a less-is-more approach. I could heal my damaged skin barrier, protect my complexion and prevent future wrinkles and blemishes, all in one step.

I knew that by combining multiple healing ingredients into a single facial oil, I could simplify my entire skincare routine. A well-formulated blend meant fewer products overall, saving me both time and money in the long run. (Hello, girl maths!) High-efficacy ingredients and fewer steps equal less waste and more savings. It was a win-win!

So I got to work. Over the course of a year, I trialled countless formulations in my kitchen, carefully fine-tuning the texture to ensure it had the perfect glideability for gua sha. I wanted it to be smooth enough to avoid tugging but not too slippery to lose control. I also wanted the formula to be low comedogenic, so it wouldn't clog pores or cause breakouts, and quick to absorb for that soft, non-greasy finish.

Fragrance-free was non-negotiable. With my sensitive skin, I knew added fragrance was a major irritant, and I wanted the oil to be gentle enough for anyone with similar struggles. But beyond that, I wanted the power of carefully selected botanical ingredients. The goal? A formula rich in vitamins A, C, E, K and more, which delivers a daily dose of nourishment and radiance.

Stress played a big role in my skincare journey, too.

Having battled stress my whole life, whether personally or in high-pressure work environments. I knew first-hand how it can wreak havoc on your skin. Stress weakens the skin barrier, causes inflammation and accelerates ageing, leaving skin red, sensitive and dull.

That's when I discovered Brahmi (*Bacopa Monnieri*), a transformative Ayurvedic ingredient that felt like the missing piece of the puzzle. Brahmi is a natural adaptogen, which means it helps the skin adapt to and recover from stress. By reducing cortisol levels, the body's stress hormones, it calms inflammation and soothes sensitivity, offering much-needed relief for troubled skin.

This remarkable ingredient also supports collagen production, enhancing elasticity and facilitating the repair of a weakened skin barrier. With its powerful antioxidant properties, Brahmi shields the skin from environmental stressors, helping to delay the visible signs of ageing. It's a true multitasker, offering both protection and rejuvenation for healthier, more resilient skin.

This discovery inspired me to dig deeper into powerful botanical actives and create a facial oil that does more than nourish, it actively works to heal stressed, menopausal and ageing skin.

The result? The award-winning Freedom Facial Oil – a thoughtfully crafted blend of ingredients designed to deliver hydration, protection and a soothing sense of calm for your complexion. It's the winner of two bronzes in the Free From Skincare Awards 2025 – in the *Leave On Facial Oil* category and a *Special Award for Labelling*. It's the formula I wish I'd had at the start of my gua sha journey, and I can't wait for it to transform your skin too.

Feedback on our facial oil from the Free From Skincare Awards was incredibly moving.

Here's what one tester had to say:

> "This feels heavenly when applied. No stinging or irritation, and it just melts into the skin. It feels rich and luxurious. I also tried using it with a gua sha, and it gave the most wonderful massage. I felt as though I'd had a professional facial. Skin looked glowing with no redness. Loved this more and more as the weeks passed. Heaven in a bottle."

There's no better compliment than being called *heaven* in a bottle – and to receive feedback like that, alongside winning awards on my first ever entry into a cosmetic competition, truly means the world. It's not just about the product. It's about the journey behind it. A reminder that you really can start with nothing but an idea, a dream and a product made with love.

This facial oil has already been a game-changer for menopausal women like Siobhan, who had long struggled with dryness and sensitivity. She shared:

> "It's instant relief, instant moisture. My skin feels deeply moisturised but never greasy – it just drinks it in. No blocked pores, no irritation and no fragrance to worry about. It feels natural and truly works."

Katy, who has dry, menopausal and itchy skin, also experienced the benefits:

> "The oil is gorgeous. It sinks into the skin perfectly, moisturising without being greasy or sticky. It's perfect over serums instead of moisturiser or on its own with my gua sha. It's even helped with my eczema patches and hasn't blocked my pores. I'm delighted with it and can see and feel a difference in my skin."

With the Freedom Facial Oil, you're not just nourishing your skin, you're giving it the care it deserves. A blend like this offers everything your skin needs: hydration, nourishment and protection, all in one bottle.

Let's break down these 10 key ingredients and why they're a game-changer for menopausal skin.

1. **Brahmi (Bacopa Monnieri).** A powerhouse Ayurvedic herb traditionally used to support stress relief and skin healing. Its antioxidant properties help calm inflammation and support skin resilience, ideal for menopausal skin prone to irritation and dullness.

2. **Jojoba Oil.** Mimics the skin's natural sebum, balancing oil production and deeply hydrating without clogging pores. Jojoba's anti-inflammatory properties soothe sensitive skin, helping with menopausal dryness and hormonal breakouts.

3. **Argan Oil.** Rich in Vitamin E and fatty acids, argan oil softens skin, boosts elasticity and protects against the effects of sun exposure. Its hydrating and antioxidant properties restore the skin barrier, leaving it smooth, plump and glowing. It's also perfect for tackling fine lines and dryness caused by menopause.

4. **Moringa Oil.** Rich in zeatin and antioxidants, this nutrient-dense oil supports skin renewal, reduces redness and helps balance uneven tone. It's particularly effective for menopausal skin dealing with blemishes, dullness and sensitivity.

5. **Prickly Pear Oil.** Packed with Vitamin K and antioxidants, prickly pear oil brightens dull skin, reduces fine lines and alleviates breakouts. It's a favourite for addressing dark circles and uneven texture, which are common concerns during menopause.

6. **Squalane.** A lightweight, plant-derived oil that deeply hydrates, strengthens the skin barrier and reduces the appearance of wrinkles. Squalane offers antioxidant benefits, protecting menopausal skin from oxidative stress and environmental damage.

7. **Passionflower Seed Oil.** Rich in essential fatty acids and antioxidants, this soothing oil helps calm and nourish dry, lacklustre skin, promoting a soft, healthy glow. It's especially beneficial for skin experiencing menopausal changes.

8. **Sea Buckthorn Oil.** A nutrient-rich oil that combats inflammation, soothes redness, and accelerates skin regeneration. High in Vitamins A and E, sea buckthorn brightens dull skin, reduces stress-related damage and provides deep nourishment to menopausal skin.

9. **Coenzyme Q10 + Vitamin E.** These antioxidants are essential for repairing and protecting the skin from environmental stressors, including UV light and pollution. Coenzyme Q10 penetrates deep into the epidermis, reducing wrinkle depth and improving firmness, which is ideal for skin experiencing loss of elasticity.

10. **Algaktiv® Zen.** A next-generation active shown in clinical testing to reduce the visible effects of stress on skin, support its natural circadian rhythm and boost radiance. It visibly smooths fine lines and revitalises tired, stressed skin.

In an effort to support my ethos of visibility and skin transparency, I wanted to make sure every consumer could understand what they're putting on their face. That's why, alongside the regulatory INCI list (the industry-standard way of listing cosmetic ingredients), we provide a simplified breakdown of every ingredient in plain English.

This commitment to clarity was recently recognised when the Freedom Facial Oil won bronze in a special labelling award, with judges praising the inclusion of the English translation as a much-needed alternative to the often confusing INCI list.

Why is this so important? Because the INCI list, while great for global standardisation, can feel like reading a foreign language to the average consumer. If a product promises to be "clean", "natural", or "eco-friendly", it's easy to assume it must be good for your skin. But that's not always the case. Understanding the ingredients puts the power back in your hands and helps you see through the marketing noise.

Here's a summary of my top four things to look out for:

1. **Ingredients are listed by concentration.** The ingredients are listed in descending order of concentration, meaning the first ingredient has the highest percentage in the formula. If a product highlights a "hero ingredient" on the label but it appears near the bottom of the list, there's likely not enough of it to make a real difference. Does the price you're paying reflect that?

2. **Water is the main ingredient.** It's common to see water listed first, but water-based formulas require preservatives to remain stable and fresh. While preservatives are essential, they can sometimes irritate sensitive skin. It's worth understanding what's keeping your product intact.

3. **Hidden fragrances are not included.** Even natural-sounding components like linalool (from lavender) can irritate sensitive or menopausal skin. These are often tucked under vague terms like "parfum" or "fragrance" near the end of the ingredient list. If you spot them, consider whether your skin truly needs them.

4. **There are no unnecessary additives, like food dyes.** Some brands add artificial colourants to give oils a golden hue, but these do nothing for your skin and may cause irritation. High-quality, effective products don't need to look flashy to deliver results.

What Makes Us Different?

Unlike many brands, we don't just throw around buzzwords. We champion full transparency. You'll know exactly what's in our products, what those ingredients do and why they're included. This builds trust and ensures you can make informed decisions about your skincare, because your skin deserves respect and not just pretty packaging.

That's why it meant so much when the *Freedom Facial Oil* was awarded bronze in a special labelling award. The judges highlighted how refreshing it was to see the plain-English translation offered alongside the INCI list, a recognition that validated our belief that ingredient clarity shouldn't be a luxury, but the standard.

Certifications also matter. Look for trustworthy symbols like organic, vegan and cruelty-free. These are excellent signs of a product's integrity. But beyond that, focus on formulas that prioritise thoughtful, high-quality ingredients that deliver real results, not just marketing fluff.

At the end of the day, skin transparency is about empowering you. By understanding the ingredients, you can choose products that genuinely care for your skin, protect your health and give you confidence in what you're using.

No gimmicks, no guesswork. Just honest, effective skincare.

Why the Freedom Facial Oil Formula Works

With the Freedom Facial Oil, less truly is more. By combining multiple healing ingredients into a single, powerful product, you simplify your routine without compromising efficacy. This thoughtful approach not only saves you time and money but also ensures your skin gets everything it needs to thrive during menopause.

As someone who has personally faced the challenges of stressed, sensitive and changing skin, I've experienced first-hand how transformative the right ingredients can be. Drawing on the ancient wisdom of Ayurveda and TCM, this carefully crafted and award-winning formula blends cultural knowledge with modern innovation, offering a truly holistic solution for menopausal skin.

Your skin deserves love, balance and gentle yet effective care during this phase of life. With its deeply nourishing and calming properties, the Freedom Facial Oil is designed to rebuild that connection between you and your skin, helping you reclaim your skin confidence.

The result? A radiant, balanced complexion and a renewed sense of self-assurance, so you can feel confident and empowered every single day, like the goddess you are.

Part 3

THE GLOW-UP PLAN

Chapter 8

THE ESSENTIAL ROLE OF NUTRITION IN NAVIGATING MENOPAUSE

Do you experience hot flushes? Mood swings? Fatigue?

Now, imagine if the foods you eat could not only ease these symptoms but also awaken the goddess within you, allowing you to move through menopause with grace, vitality and power. Nutrition isn't just about sustenance; it is sacred nourishment, a way to honour your body and embrace this transformative phase of life. The right foods don't just fuel you; they heal you, balance your energy and reconnect you with your divine feminine wisdom.

In Traditional Chinese Medicine (TCM) and Japanese nutrition, food is regarded as medicine.

As Hippocrates, the father of medicine, famously stated,

"Let food be thy medicine and medicine be thy food."

These ancient traditions have long emphasised that what you eat directly influences your body's balance, health and vitality. By embracing this wisdom and making intentional choices, you can manage your symptoms, nourish your body and reclaim control over your wellbeing.

That's right, you literally have the power to become symptom-free.

Sounds amazing, right?

Food as Your Ally

What you eat during menopause shapes everything, from your energy levels and radiant glow to your emotional harmony and the way you experience this transition. Around the world, cultures have long recognised the profound connection between food and overall wellbeing.

In particular, women in Japan, China and Korea report fewer and less intense menopausal symptoms compared to women in the West. The secret? Their diet.

But this isn't just about what you eat, it's about the energy of the food itself. TCM teaches that food carries an energetic signature, profoundly influencing the body's balance. You have the power to turn down your internal "thermostat" by choosing cooling, *yin*-nourishing foods – nature's own air-conditioning. For all the radiant goddesses experiencing hot flushes, this wisdom is going to be a game-changer!

Rooted in a holistic understanding of balance, Asian dietary traditions focus on supporting hormonal harmony, replenishing deep nourishment and regulating body temperature. This isn't just about symptom relief, it's about stepping into your power and embracing menopause as a time of renewal and transformation.

Japanese women, celebrated for their longevity and graceful ageing, embody this philosophy. Their traditional diet is rich in nutrient-dense, hormone-supportive foods that work in harmony with the body rather than against it. They don't resist change; they flow with it, honouring the body's natural rhythms.

Let's explore how these sacred principles can empower you to navigate menopause with strength, wisdom and radiance.

Three Core Principles for Menopause Nutrition

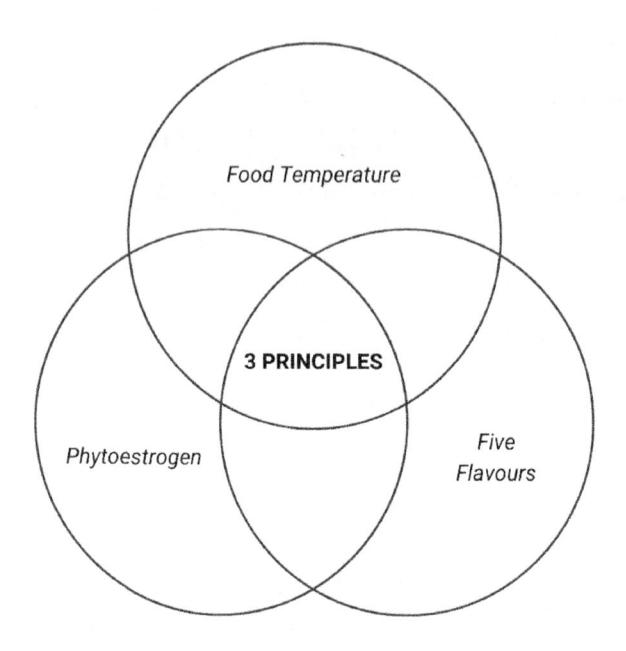

```
         Food Temperature

  Phytoestrogen    3 PRINCIPLES    Five
                                  Flavours
```

Integrating these three core principles into designing every meal is a game-changer for menopause and overall wellbeing.

1. **Food Temperatures.** Balance foods that cool or warm your body to regulate temperature fluctuations.

2. **Five Flavours.** Include sweet, sour, pungent, bitter and salty flavours to maximise nutrients and enjoyment.

3. **Phytoestrogens.** Incorporate plant-based oestrogen-like compounds to support hormonal balance (e.g. soy).

Let's explore these principles in more detail.

Food Temperatures

Have you ever thought about how the foods you eat could affect your body's internal "thermostat"? This isn't about the temperature of your meal when served, but the effect certain foods have on whether your body heats up or cools down. During menopause, fluctuating oestrogen levels can lead to noticeable changes in body temperature, often experienced as hot flushes. Here's where understanding food temperatures can be an absolute game-changer.

Incorporating cooling "cold foods" into your diet is essential if your body tends to run hot. Think of a hot summer's day when you instinctively reach for a slice of watermelon because it's refreshing, hydrating and naturally cooling. The same principle applies to managing hot flushes during menopause. Cooling foods can calm your body from the inside out, acting as a natural air conditioner.

However, balance is key. TCM teaches that relying too heavily on cold foods can inhibit digestion, potentially leading to an upset stomach. Instead, aim to mix cold and warm foods in your meals for the perfect balance and maximum benefit.

Some of the best cooling foods to include are cucumber, celery, daikon radish, cabbage, mung beans, pak choi, cauliflower, carrots and romaine lettuce. Cooling fruits like watermelon, grapefruit, apples, pears and apricots are also excellent choices.

Make it a habit to eat at least two servings of these cold foods daily to help regulate your body temperature and keep those hot flushes at bay.

When you pair this approach with warm, digestion-supporting foods such as ginger or quinoa, you create a balanced meal that works harmoniously with your body. By incorporating this principle into your diet, you're not just managing symptoms, you're taking control of your menopause journey in a way that's natural, effective and empowering.

Five Flavours

Imagine creating meals that aren't just delicious but also work wonders for your health. That's the magic of balancing the five core flavours: sweet, salty, sour, bitter, and pungent. This balance is an integral principle of Asian diets. Not only does this approach make every bite a sensory delight, but it also ensures your body receives a wide spectrum of nutrients, with each flavour delivering unique health benefits. If you're navigating menopause, this method is something you absolutely have to try!

For menopausal women, bitter foods may be especially beneficial because they naturally cool the body, making them a fantastic ally in easing hot flushes and night sweats. Bitter foods also play a powerful role in digestion. When you taste something bitter, it's like sending a wake-up call to your digestive system. Your saliva production increases, and the hormone gastrin is released, stimulating the movement of your intestines and allowing your body to absorb maximum nutrition from your meals. In Japan, for instance, drinking vinegar, a sour and slightly bitter tonic rich in gut-friendly acetic acid, is a common pre-meal ritual that aids digestion and boosts metabolism.

During my time in Bali, I encountered a remarkable healer in Ubud who swore by the daily ritual of drinking apple cider vinegar mixed with water. Curious, I asked, "Why?" The healer informed me that it aids digestion, detoxifies the body and brings mental clarity. This healer had been following the practice for years and considered it essential for clear thinking. What intrigued me most was how the concept of consuming bitter foods for health benefits transcends cultures, from the Balinese tradition to the wisdom of the Japanese.

Here's how the five flavours translate to everyday foods:

For pungent foods, think of foods like ginger, onion and chilli peppers. These stimulate circulation, invigorate the body and improve energy levels.

For sweet foods, naturally sweet foods such as honey, rice, wheat and pears provide a sense of comfort and support energy balance.

For sour foods, tomatoes, oranges and plums aid digestion, enhance metabolism and cleanse the liver.

For bitter foods, cooling foods like kale, parsley, watercress and green tea are your best friends for managing hot flushes and boosting digestion.

For salty foods, pickles, sauerkraut and seaweed provide essential minerals, support hydration and improve adrenal health.

Why is balancing these flavours so transformative during menopause?

Each flavour brings its own strengths, but together they create harmony in the body. Sweet and salty balance your energy, while sour and pungent stimulate circulation and digestion. Bitter offers the cooling and detoxifying effects your body craves during menopause. By combining all five flavours, you'll not only craft meals that excite your taste buds but also support your body in a profound way.

When planning your meals, it may be beneficial to include all five flavours, giving special attention to bitter foods. They can help turn down the heat during hot flushes, support your digestive health and even help regulate mood swings. It's time to embrace this holistic approach. You'll be amazed by how vibrant and empowered you feel!

Phytoestrogens

Have you ever wished for a natural way to manage the rollercoaster of menopausal symptoms? Enter phytoestrogens, which are powerful plant compounds that mimic oestrogen in the body. These incredible nutrients can help alleviate symptoms like hot flushes, night sweats, vaginal dryness, mood swings and even the loss of bone density – all challenges brought on by hormonal changes during menopause.

The secret lies in cultures like Japan and China, where soy, an ingredient rich in phytoestrogens, features prominently in daily diets. Women in these regions consistently report fewer and less severe menopausal symptoms compared to their Western counterparts, and it's no coincidence. Studies reveal that phytoestrogens, especially isoflavones found in soy, can significantly reduce the frequency and intensity of hot flushes.

Here's how you can bring the benefits of phytoestrogens to your table:

Soy Isoflavones (Superfood)

Nourishing Suggestions: Tofu, tempeh, miso, soy milk, edamame

Why It May Work: Isoflavones are the most potent phytoestrogens, acting like a natural oestrogen substitute to balance hormonal fluctuations.

Choose organic, non-GMO soy products for maximum benefits. You can also opt for fermented soy, like miso or natto, to support gut health while reaping additional nutritional perks. You can also add tofu to stir-fries, enjoy miso soup or snack on edamame for an easy daily boost of isoflavones.

Flaxseeds (Fibre)

Nourishing Suggestions: Ground flaxseeds or flaxseed oil

Why It May Work: Flaxseeds contain lignans, another type of phytoestrogen, which help with hormone balance and support cardiovascular health.

Sprinkle ground flaxseeds over your morning porridge, blend them into smoothies or use flaxseed oil as a salad dressing for an easy oestrogen boost.

Legumes (Plant Protein)

Nourishing Suggestions: Chickpeas, lentils and beans

Why It May Work: Packed with phytoestrogens, plant protein and fibre, legumes not only balance hormones but also promote digestive health and stable energy levels.

Add lentils to soups, whip up hummus with chickpeas or enjoy a hearty bean salad for a satisfying and hormone-friendly meal.

Whole Grains (Fibre)

Nourishing Suggestions: Oats, barley, rye and wheat

Why It May Work: Whole grains are rich in lignans and other phytoestrogenic compounds that promote heart health and support digestion.

Swap white bread for whole-grain options, try a warm bowl of barley risotto or enjoy porridge oats topped with fruits and nuts for a wholesome, hormone-balancing start to your day.

Nuts and Seeds (Healthy Fats, Fibres, Vitamins and Minerals)

Nourishing Suggestions: Sesame seeds, sunflower seeds and walnuts

Why It May Work: High in lignans and healthy fats, nuts and seeds help regulate hormones and reduce inflammation.

Snack on walnuts, sprinkle sesame seeds over stir-fries or add sunflower seeds to your salads for an effortless phytoestrogen boost.

Fruits and Vegetables (Antioxidants, Vitamins and Minerals)

Nourishing Suggestions: Apples, berries, carrots, broccoli and spinach

Why It May Work: These foods provide a moderate amount of phytoestrogens alongside antioxidants, vitamins and minerals that support overall health.

Enjoy apples as a midday snack, add berries to your yoghurt and include broccoli or spinach in your evening meals to maximise their nutritional value.

Incorporating phytoestrogen-rich foods into your diet is a holistic way to nurture your entire body. These foods support bone health, heart health and even skin vitality. They are your natural allies in bringing balance to your hormones while keeping your meals diverse, delicious and deeply nourishing.

Ready to get started? You could try adding at least one phytoestrogen-rich food to each meal. Whether it's a spoonful of flaxseeds in your breakfast, a serving of tofu in your lunch or a handful of nuts for a snack, these small steps may make a world of difference. Let food be your medicine and reclaim your wellbeing one bite at a time.

Spotlight on Key Foods

Carrots

Carrots are a powerhouse for menopausal health. Rich in beta-carotene, they convert into Vitamin A in the body, a nutrient essential for skin rejuvenation. Vitamin A promotes collagen production, which enhances skin elasticity, reduces the appearance of fine lines and helps maintain a radiant complexion – a welcome benefit during menopause, when skin can become drier and less supple. Carrots also contain antioxidants that combat free radicals, helping to reduce inflammation and protect your skin from premature ageing.

Enjoy them raw, roasted or blended into soups to nourish your body from the inside out.

Cruciferous Vegetables

When it comes to supporting hormonal health, cruciferous vegetables like broccoli, cauliflower, kale and brussel sprouts are true champions. These vegetables are rich in indole-3-carbinol and sulforaphane, compounds that aid in oestrogen metabolism by helping the body process and eliminate excess hormones. This is particularly important during menopause, when hormonal imbalances can intensify symptoms like hot flushes and mood swings.

Beyond their hormone-regulating benefits, cruciferous vegetables are packed with antioxidants that combat inflammation and oxidative stress, which can accelerate ageing and lead to chronic conditions. They're also high in fibre, supporting gut health and improving digestion, which is key for maintaining overall wellness during this phase of life.

Try steaming, stir-frying, or roasting these vegetables to bring out their natural flavours and maximise their health benefits.

Take Charge of Your Menopause Journey

Your diet is a powerful tool for navigating menopause. By balancing cooling and warming foods, incorporating all five flavours and embracing phytoestrogens, you may be able to alleviate symptoms, nourish your body and thrive during this phase of life.

So, why wait? Start today. Fill your plate with foods that support, empower and nourish you, inside and out.

Here's a glimpse of your ultimate goddess guide to nourishment. For 50 powerful, healthy ingredients designed to support you through menopause, turn to Appendix 2 at the back of this book.

You could take this cheat sheet with you to the supermarket like the empowered queen you are, because balancing your body's internal temperatures through food is an act of self-love. Own this journey. Claim your power. You are radiant, you are strong, and you are in control.

No.	Food	Food Temperature	Flavour	Benefit
1	Apples	Cool	Sweet	Antioxidant-rich, supports digestion and balances meals
2	Apple Cider Vinegar	Cool	Sour	Aids digestion, supports gut health and helps balance blood sugar levels
3	Aubergine	Cool	Bitter	High in fibre, supports heart health and helps with oestrogen metabolism
4	Avocado	Neutral	Sweet	Rich in healthy fats, it supports skin health and hormone regulation

No.	Food	Food Temperature	Flavour	Benefit
5	Barley	Neutral	Sweet	Cooling grain aids digestion and supports heart health
6	Berries	Cool	Sweet	High in antioxidants, supports brain health and reduces inflammation
7	Brocolli	Neutral	Bitter	Supports oestrogen metabolism and detoxification, high in antioxidants
8	Brussel Sprouts	Neutral	Bitter	High in antioxidants, supports hormonal health and detoxification
9	Cabbage	Cold	Sweet	High in fibre and antioxidants, supports digestion and reduces inflammation
10	Carrots	Neutral	Sweet	High in beta-carotene, it supports skin health and boosts collagen production

For the full checklist, see Appendix 2 (50 Essential Ingredients for Menopause-Friendly Meals) at the back of the book.

Embracing East Asian Eating Practices to Ease Menopause

Across cultures like Japan and Korea, meals are beautifully balanced, incorporating vegetables, protein and carbohydrates in a thoughtful sequence designed to maximise digestion, maintain blood sugar stability and support hormonal harmony.

Following this order – vegetables first, protein second and carbohydrates last – can enhance satiety, regulate energy and ease menopausal symptoms naturally.

Here's how you could adopt these practices into your daily meals, with examples inspired by both Japanese and Korean traditions.

A gentle reminder: The information in this chapter is shared as general guidance and inspiration. For advice tailored to your unique needs, we recommend consulting with a qualified nutritionist, dietitian or an appropriate professional.

Breakfast: Energise Your Morning

You could start your day with a balanced and nutrient-dense Japanese-inspired breakfast.

Nourishing Suggestions

- **Miso soup**. Rich in fermented soy, miso provides gut-friendly probiotics and phytoestrogens that mimic oestrogen, helping to reduce hot flushes.

- **Spinach namul (Korean sesame spinach).** This lightly seasoned side dish is rich in calcium, iron and magnesium, making it an excellent support for bone health during menopause. It's wonderfully simple to prepare: Briefly boil spinach for a minute, then plunge it into cold water to stop the cooking. Squeeze out all excess water, then mix with a tablespoon of roasted sesame oil, a splash of soy sauce, and a teaspoon of finely chopped garlic. Chill before serving.

This is one of my all-time favourite side dishes. There's always a container of it in my fridge. I often eat a couple of spoonfuls before meals or reach for it as a nourishing snack when I'm feeling peckish.

- **Grilled salmon or a boiled egg**. Provides protein and omega-3s to reduce inflammation and ease joint pain.

Why It May Work

This combination delivers gut-friendly probiotics, hormone-supportive phytoestrogens and anti-inflammatory omega-3s while adhering to the optimal eating order.

Breakfast Alternatives

- **Chia seed pudding.** High in fibre, omega-3s, and antioxidants, this pudding stabilises blood sugar and combats oxidative stress.

  Ingredients: Almond milk (or coconut milk), chia seeds, and a drizzle of honey. Optional: top with your favourite fruit or matcha powder.

- **Vegetable rice porridge (okayu or juk).** Easy to digest and naturally soothing, this warming breakfast supports gut health, mood stability and gentle energy.

  Ingredients: Cooked short-grain rice simmered with water or bone broth, top with vegetables of your choice, a soft egg and a drizzle of sesame oil

- **Tamago sushi-inspired omelette wrap.** A protein-rich, portable option with phytoestrogens and minerals from nori.

  Ingredients: A thin Japanese-style omelette (tamago), rolled around sautéed spinach and a sprinkle of nori flakes.

Lunch: Light and Nourishing

Midday meals in Japan are often light yet nutrient-packed, designed to sustain energy without causing a mid-afternoon slump.

Nourishing Suggestions

- **Silken tofu bowl with edamame and crispy onions.** Light yet satisfying, this high-protein, calcium-rich bowl supports muscle function, bone health, and hormonal balance.

  Ingredients: Silken tofu topped with shelled edamame, a drizzle of sesame oil and low-sodium soy sauce, finished with chopped spring onions, crispy onions, black sesame seeds, and a pinch of togarashi (optional) for heat.

- **Grilled tofu, chicken or mackerel.** High in protein and phytoestrogens, aiding muscle repair and hormone balance.

- **Pickled vegetables (tsukemono) or kimchi.** Fermented foods to support digestion and gut health. Add this as a side to your lunch to aid in digestion.

- **A side of soba noodles or quinoa.** Provides slow-releasing carbohydrates for steady energy.

Why It May Work

Starting with fibre-rich seaweed and vegetables primes digestion, while protein keeps you full and carbohydrates round out the meal without spiking blood sugar.

Lunch Alternatives

- **Quinoa salad with edamame and wakame.** A protein-rich, gluten-free option with gut-supporting minerals from seaweed.

  Ingredients: Quinoa, shelled edamame, wakame seaweed, cherry tomatoes and a light sesame dressing. Optional: Add grilled chicken for extra protein.

- **Steamed fish with ginger and spring onions.** Light, aromatic, and nourishing, this dish is rich in lean protein and anti-inflammatory compounds, making it perfect for balanced blood sugar and sustained energy.

  Ingredients: Steamed white fish (such as cod or sea bass), julienned ginger, spring onions, tamari or light soy sauce, sesame oil, steamed bok choy and a small serving of brown rice.

- **Vegetable and mushroom udon soup.** A comforting and nutrient-dense soup offering antioxidants and complex carbohydrates.

  Ingredients: A light dashi broth with udon noodles, shiitake mushrooms, carrots and baby spinach.

Dinner: Restore and Rejuvenate

Evening meals are an opportunity to relax and replenish, with foods that support restful sleep and recovery.

Nourishing Suggestions

- **Vegetable stir-fry with bok choy, mushrooms, and carrots.** Packed with antioxidants and fibre to combat oxidative stress and support digestion.

- **Grilled chicken breast.** Rich in protein and omega-3s to aid muscle repair and cognitive health.

- **Miso soup with wakame.** A comforting end to the day, promoting gut health and hydration.

- **A small portion of sweet potato.** Provides complex carbohydrates to restore glycogen stores.

Why It May Work

This meal emphasises anti-inflammatory and nutrient-dense foods while ensuring a balanced intake of all macronutrients.

Dinner Alternatives

- **Grilled miso-glazed eggplant with sesame seeds.** High in phytonutrients and minerals, this dish supports bone and hormonal health.

  Ingredients: Eggplant brushed with a miso glaze and sprinkled with toasted sesame seeds, served with a side of steamed bok choy.

- **Kimchi jigae (spicy kimchi stew).** A warming, probiotic-rich stew that supports gut health, reduces inflammation, and helps regulate hormones, especially beneficial during menopause.

  Ingredients: Aged kimchi simmered with tofu cubes, onion, garlic, gochugaru (Korean chilli flakes), a splash of soy sauce, and a touch of sesame oil. Optional additions include mushrooms, zucchini, or a small amount of sliced pork or tempeh for extra protein.

- **Miso salmon with steamed vegetables.** Packed with omega-3s and phytoestrogens to support brain health and hormone balance.

  Ingredients: Salmon fillet marinated in miso, grilled until tender. Served with steamed broccoli and carrots.

- **Vegetable katsu curry.** a satisfying, plant-based dinner rich in fibre and essential nutrients.

    Ingredients: Breaded and baked slices of aubergine or sweet potato served with a mild curry sauce and a side of brown rice.

The Science Behind the Veg → Protein → Carbs Sequence

Starting with vegetables like high-fibre vegetables like spinach, seaweed or broccoli, reduce the glycaemic impact of carbohydrates and promote digestion.

Then, moving to protein sources such as fish, tofu or eggs stabilise blood sugar and provide essential amino acids for muscle repair and energy.

Ending with carbohydrates and consuming complex carbohydrates like brown rice or sweet potatoes last prevents blood sugar spikes and supports steady energy levels.

Benefits of This Approach

   Improved blood sugar control. Prevents energy crashes and cravings.

   Enhanced digestion. Fibre primes the gut, while protein digests effectively without interference.

Balanced hormonal response. Stable blood sugar aids insulin regulation, reducing menopausal weight gain.

Tips for Success

Incorporate soy daily. Add miso, tofu, or soy milk to your meals for phytoestrogen benefits.

Sip green tea. Replace sugary drinks with antioxidant-rich green tea to combat oxidative stress and promote relaxation.

Experiment with seaweed. Sprinkle nori on salads or use wakame in soups to boost mineral intake.

Mindful eating. Slow down, savour each bite and eat until 80% full. This is a practice known as *hara hachi bu*.

By embracing these Japanese and Korean-inspired principles, you are creating sacred rituals of nourishment, designed to soothe your symptoms, restore balance and elevate your wellbeing. Every bite becomes an opportunity to honour your body, to listen to what it needs, and to step into your goddess power with intention.

Allow the wisdom of Japanese and Korean cuisine to guide you as you take charge of your health with grace, intuition and confidence. Start by incorporating cooling, hormone-supportive foods into your meals. Tune in to your body's cravings and honour them with nourishment that energises, heals and empowers you.

When planning your meals, you could consult Appendix 2 (50 Essential Ingredients for Menopause-Friendly Meals), because a goddess feeds her body with wisdom, love and intention.

Chapter 9
DESIGNING YOUR ROUTINE

This chapter is about more than just organisation. It's about stepping into your divine power and creating a structure that supports your success, nurtures your wellbeing and allows you to move through life with ease and confidence. A woman aligned with her inner strength doesn't simply react to life; she takes control, sets intentions and moves with purpose. Imagine how empowering it would feel to have a routine attuned to your highest self that helps you manage menopause with grace, feeling strong, radiant and fully in charge of your body and mind.

Routines are so much more than a schedule; they are a sacred act of self-care, a daily commitment to honouring yourself and your needs. They become especially vital when life feels unpredictable, when your body is changing and when emotions run high.

A well-structured rhythm becomes your anchor, offering stability and a sense of calm amidst transformation.

Menopause is not a loss; it's an awakening, a time to reconnect with yourself on a deeper level. But to do that, you must set the foundation, which is a routine that supports, strengthens and uplifts you.

True empowerment begins with mindset. A woman who knows her worth understands that real power comes from consistency, dedication and trust in the process. The key is to be flexible, intuitive and patient. Creating a new routine, especially from scratch, is a journey of self-discovery. It won't happen overnight, but with intentional action and self-belief, it becomes second nature. Think of it as crafting a new rhythm for your life, one that aligns with your most radiant energy and allows you to move through each day feeling supported and capable.

We've explored powerful tools to incorporate into your self-care rituals: skincare to nourish your glow, gua sha to relieve tension and enhance circulation, and nutrition to fuel your body from within. Each practice is a piece of your wellness mosaic. By weaving them together, you create a personalised, soul-nurturing routine that not only meets your physical needs but also elevates your entire being.

As you design your routine, embrace it as a living, breathing expression of your highest energy, something that evolves with you and always serves your greater good. Some days will call for deep rest and reflection; others may call for movement and expansion. The beauty of a well-crafted routine is that it flows with you, adapting to the natural rhythms of your life.

Step into this process with excitement, embrace the shifts and celebrate every small win. You are not just building a routine; you're creating a powerful foundation for the next chapter of your life. You are rising into your fullest potential, glowing through change and moving forward with clarity, strength and confidence.

Unlocking Your Routine – My Best-Kept Secret!

Let's talk about planning. It's the cornerstone of any successful routine. Whether you're pursuing your dream, building a new habit or navigating a big life transition, planning transforms overwhelm into action. It's not just about writing down tasks; it's about setting clear objectives, breaking them into manageable steps and crafting a roadmap to achieve them. Once you start doing this, you'll feel unstoppable.

I met Marie on a ThetaHealing course, and we instantly clicked. My favourite question to ask anyone I meet is, "If you could do anything in the world, where money wasn't an option, what would it be?" She shared that she has this amazing goal of teaching yoga with a twist, a combination of yoga with healing. I asked when she was planning on pursuing her dream, and she replied as most people do: "Someday."

Remember, "someday" isn't a day of the week. It's not a quantifiable measure of time.

We discussed the fears of becoming an entrepreneur and stepping into the spotlight, and the power of planning.

"It *is* possible to manage it all and more," I said encouragingly.

"How did you do it?" She asked curiously.

I shared the power of planning, the 12-week calendar technique and my steps to achieving your goals in a short space of time. It is so important to set mini-actionable goals and carve out time in your schedule to achieve them. It's easier said than done, but I also talked about ways to navigate resistance when it crops up, because it will!

How you turn "someday" into tomorrow is to let go of perfection. Perfection isn't a standard of excellence.

When it comes to setting goals and achieving them, we need to reframe our mindset to "progress, not perfection." Read that again.

Now, Marie is working on finishing off her yoga certification, juggling her job and preparing to launch her yoga classes to clients, and I'm so excited to see how she transforms her dreams into a reality.

Here's the thing: Planning is my superpower. Over the last three years, I've accomplished what seemed impossible – qualifying as a solicitor, launching a skincare business, becoming a certified Theta Healer, travelling on adventurous holidays and, most recently, writing this book. People often ask me, "How do you manage to fit it all in?"

The answer is simple: Great planning leads to great results.

Today, I'm letting you in on my best-kept secret. I can't believe I'm sharing this because it's that good.

Step 1: Pick No More Than Three Goals

Let's start with a golden rule: Less is more. Why three goals? Focusing on just three allows you to channel your energy effectively, avoid feeling overwhelmed and stay motivated. It's like juggling. You can easily manage three balls, but try to juggle four and it all falls apart.

When I worked as a paralegal at a demanding US law firm, I had three ambitious goals:

1. Perform at my best in a high-pressure job.
2. Pass my Solicitors' Qualifying Exams (SQE).
3. Lay the groundwork for launching my skincare business, SHANTI[3].

These were bold goals, but having only three meant I could give each one the attention it needed. It also gave me the confidence to say *no* to things that didn't align with my priorities.

When setting your own goals, make sure they're meaningful to you and aligned with what you truly want, not what you think you *should* do.

Step 2: Identify Challenges and Resistance Points

Once you've set your goals, it's time for some honest reflection. What might stop you from achieving them? This step requires genuine self-awareness, as it involves confronting your excuses and fears.

This can be difficult as our brains are naturally wired to prioritise safety and comfort. Change feels uncomfortable because it pushes us into the unknown. Your mind will come up with all sorts of reasons why you can't do something: I'm too busy, I'm too tired, I'll start next week. Sound familiar? During menopause, life is already busy with responsibilities – putting yourself first often feels like a luxury you can't afford.

For me, the biggest challenge was time – a problem that I'm sure many of you can relate to. I felt time-poor. I was working long hours at the law firm, often late into the night, which made studying during the week unrealistic. Trying to cram everything into the weekend wasn't sustainable either.

The solution? A time management makeover. I completely restructured my schedule and negotiated a four-day work week for six months, freeing up Fridays for a dedicated 10-hour study day. Sundays became my "split" day. Mornings were for self-care and relaxation, and afternoons were for working on my business, like designing packaging and planning the launch strategy.

This deliberate approach gave each goal its own space in my life. By breaking the week into focused blocks, I felt less overwhelmed and more in control.

If you're serious about starting a new routine, you have to make room for it in your life. We always make time for what's truly important to us, so be honest about your priorities and carve out the time you need.

Step 3: Build Accountability

Motivation isn't a constant; it ebbs and flows. On the days when you're feeling drained or unmotivated, accountability is your secret weapon.

I knew that studying alone, especially after a long week, would be tough. To stay on track, I partnered with an online study buddy based in Saudi Arabia. Despite the time difference, we motivated each other, shared ideas and kept each other accountable. Having someone to check in with made studying feel less daunting, more structured and even enjoyable.

Here's the crucial part: Your accountability partner needs to share your commitment to their own goals. Your friend might not be the right person if they're not on the same wavelength. Look for someone who values consistency and shares your drive for personal growth and improvement.

This method works brilliantly for other areas as well, like fitness. If you're trying to build an exercise routine, consider joining a class or finding a workout buddy. Whether it's a Pilates session or a brisk walk with a friend, knowing someone is counting on you helps you show up, even when you don't feel like it.

Step 4: Beat Procrastination with Rewards

We all procrastinate, especially when faced with tasks we dread. For me, that was studying dry topics like wills and estate law or property law (no offence to anyone who loves it). So, to tackle procrastination, I adopted a simple reward system.

Just like a child earning gold stars, I gave myself a treat every time I completed a task or stuck to my plan each week. My rewards weren't sugary snacks (though tempting!) but things that nurtured my wellbeing.

Here's what my reward system looked like:

- **Daily "mini" treats** like a 30-minute walk, a luxurious face mask or enjoying an episode of my favourite show.

- **Weekly treats** like a long bath, an evening off with friends or taking a leisurely nap.

- **Big rewards** like something exciting to look forward to as I worked through the tough weeks. For example, after my exams, I planned a celebratory trip.

This approach made tasks feel less intimidating and gave me something positive to focus on. However, I limited this system to a six-week period. Why? Because by then, I knew I'd built enough momentum to keep going without needing external incentives. Seeing real progress became the ultimate motivator.

My pro tip for rewarding yourself would be to choose rewards that genuinely support your health and happiness. While it's tempting to treat yourself to sugary snacks or late nights, these don't always align with your bigger goals. Think long baths, quality time with loved ones or an indulgent skincare ritual instead.

Step 5: Create a Visual Plan (Macro Perspective)

You've identified your goals, challenges and solutions, and now it's time to bring your vision to life! Imagine holding the blueprint for your success in your hands. That's what we're about to create. Grab an A3-sized 12-week calendar (a physical one, as I swear it makes a difference), and let's map your journey from where you are today to where you want to be.

Why 12 weeks? This timeframe is a game-changer. It's long enough to see real progress yet short enough to stay focused. Unlike vague, year-long goals, 12-week plans demand action here and now.

Trust me, you'll accomplish more in 12 weeks than you would chasing yearly targets. Plus, seeing your entire plan laid out in front of you provides clarity and a sense of commitment that's hard to beat.

Here's the best part: this system works anytime. No need to wait for January 1st. Start when it feels right for you, though beginning on the first of a month can be especially motivating, and it looks so satisfying on your calendar!

This 12-week plan is your macro perspective or the bird's-eye view of your journey. It's crucial because it keeps your *"why"* front and centre. On tough days when you're tempted to quit, this visual plan will remind you of your purpose, your progress and what's still ahead. Place it somewhere prominent, such as in your kitchen, office or even your bedroom, and let it inspire you daily.

With your big-picture plan in place, it's time to focus on the details. Let's dive into the day-to-day strategy.

Step 6: Day-to-Day Planning (Micro Perspective)

Now let's shift from the big picture to the daily grind. This is about creating a micro perspective, or your day-to-day commitment to your goals.

Let me share an invaluable perspective I learned as a lawyer: Lawyers bill their time in 6-minute increments. Every 6 minutes equals 0.1 units of chargeable time. At the end of each day, these units are inputted, creating a clear record of where every moment went. Annoying admin? Yes. However, it taught me an invaluable lesson: Time is a valuable currency.

Every moment counts, and when you start assigning value to your time, you'll make it work harder for you.

Here's the breakdown:

Time	Units
6 minutes	0.1
30 minutes	0.5
1 hour	1.0
24 hours	24.0

You, me, everyone – we all have 24 hours in a day. The question is, how are you spending yours? To build a routine that works, you first need to calculate your actionable active hours.

Calculating Your Actionable Active Hours

To use your time effectively, you first need to understand how much of it you can actively control. These are your actionable active hours, or the blocks of time you can allocate to your goals after accounting for essential commitments.

Here's how to calculate them:

1. **Start with 24 hours.** Everyone begins the day with the same amount of time.

2. **Subtract hours spent sleeping.** Aim for 7 to 9 hours of quality rest each night. Sleep isn't a luxury; it's a non-negotiable investment in your wellbeing.

3. **Subtract work hours.** Include your commute if applicable.

4. **Account for daily responsibilities.** Cooking, cleaning, childcare and errands – these are part of life but shouldn't dominate your schedule.

5. **What's left is yours.** This is your time to shape, filled with potential to move closer to your goals.

For an example calculation: if you sleep for 8 hours, work and commute for 10 hours, and spend 2 hours on household chores, you're left with 4 hours of actionable active time.

A Day in the Life: Sunday Schedule Example

Let's bring this to life with a practical example. Imagine you're planning a balanced and fulfilling Sunday:

Time	Activity
9:30 am	Wakeup
9:40 am	Get ready for Pilates
9:50 am	Walk to class
10:00 am	Pilates (2 hours)
12:05 pm	Walk home
12:15 pm	Shower
12:30 pm	Skincare routine with gua sha
12:45 pm	Get dressed and apply makeup
1:00 pm	Commute to lunch
1:45 pm	Dim Sum lunch with a friend
3:15 pm	Shopping
4:30 pm	Cinema
7:00 pm	Dinner
8:30 pm	Commute home
9:00 pm	Unwind
9:30 pm	Watch TV
10:00 pm	Evening skincare routine
10:15 pm	Bedtime

This example demonstrates a balanced day that includes self-care, fitness, socialising and downtime. Planning this way might feel daunting, but stick with me.

Plotting out your time helps you see where your hours are going. If life throws a curveball (as it often does), it's not a disaster. You simply adjust.

Practical Goal Setting

When setting goals, language matters. How you frame your goals can determine whether you achieve them.

For example, instead of saying "I want to lose 10kg," which subconsciously focuses on losing, try framing it as: "I feel healthier by doing three strength-training classes and three Pilates sessions every week for 12 weeks."

This goal is positive, actionable and measurable. This approach shifts the focus from a fixed outcome to an ongoing process, which is more motivating and sustainable.

Once your goals are clear, break them down:

Plan your schedule. Use a 12-week calendar to allocate time for each class.

Book your classes. Add them to your phone calendar and set reminders.

Track your progress. Tick off completed activities on your printed 12-week calendar. Physical progress tracking is incredibly satisfying!

Adapt when needed. If you miss a session, don't panic. Revisit your schedule and look for lower-value time slots (like 30 minutes of TV) to make up for it.

Flexibility is key, but so is accountability.

Time is Your Most Precious Resource

In law, we place a monetary value on every minute of our day. When you start viewing time as your most valuable currency, everything changes. Waiting for perpetually late friends? Engaging in draining relationships? Scrolling aimlessly through your phone? Those are hidden costs you can't afford.

If you truly value your time, you'll invest it wisely. This means allocating time to what matters: yourself, your goals and your happiness. This mindset transforms how you approach relationships, work and self-care. It's not just about fitting goals into your day; it's about making your routine a powerful framework for the life you want.

Menopause: A Time of Renewal

Menopause is a time of reinvention. Maybe your kids are grown, your career is evolving or you're exploring new passions and spirituality.

Take this opportunity to reassess how you spend your time. Is your routine supporting your growth and happiness? If not, it's time for a refresh. Align your routine with the life you truly want.

Here's how to create a routine that's both achievable and inspiring:

Print a 12-week calendar. Go A3 size or bigger (the bigger the better!).

Colour-code your goals. Use a different colour for each focus area (e.g. fitness can be blue, self-care can be green and healthy eating can be pink).

Add tasks to your phone calendar. Include reminders, even for short activities like a 6-minute gua sha session.

Track your progress. Tick off tasks on your printed calendar. Celebrate small wins to stay motivated!

Keep your calendar visible. Display your 12-week calendar where you'll see it daily. Let it inspire and motivate you.

With these tools, you're ready to create a routine that empowers you to thrive. Don't think about it as just ticking off goals. Instead, think of it as making this stage of your life joyful, fulfilling and uniquely yours.

Trusting the Process

Implementing a new routine is not just an adjustment; it is a declaration of your power. You are no longer drifting through change; you're embracing it, shaping it and transforming it into an opportunity for self-mastery. Menopause is a sacred evolution, and by crafting a routine that nurtures both body and soul, you step fully into your divine feminine energy, feeling balanced, radiant and in control.

It's tempting to crave instant transformation, but true growth is a slow unfolding, not a rushed destination. Trusting the process means believing in the magic of your consistent efforts, knowing that every small act of self-care, every mindful choice, is leading you closer to harmony, strength and vitality.

Your body is transitioning into its most intuitive, powerful form. Some days will be filled with fire and energy, while others call for softness and reflection. The key is to honour each phase with grace. Don't resist the shifts. Instead, flow with them. Let your routine become a sanctuary, not a rigid list of tasks, but a flexible, sacred structure that holds you steady as life ebbs and flows.

View this transformation as the small, intentional rituals woven into your daily life that create lasting magic. A morning gratitude practice, a few minutes of deep breathing, a nourishing meal that fuels your body and spirit – these are not minor acts. They are the building blocks of your goddess power.

Patience: The Secret to Thriving

Lasting growth isn't forced, it's nurtured. Instead of chasing perfection, honour the process. Patience is one of your greatest tools. It allows you to show up fully, even when progress feels slow, and to trust that meaningful change is already underway.

Practice patience by setting realistic intentions. Success isn't about flawless execution. It's about consistency. Sustainable, soul-aligned habits will serve you far longer than rigid expectations.

And when life interrupts your rhythm, don't crumble. Recalibrate – flow with the change. Every challenge is an invitation to tune in, listen and adapt with wisdom.

Lastly, celebrate every win. Did you show yourself love today? Did you rest when you needed to? Did you breathe, move, or nourish yourself in some way? Honour those moments. They are milestones on your path to full embodiment.

Progress Over Perfection

Not every day will be seamless, but every day is an opportunity to show up for yourself. Your routine is not a chore. It is an act of devotion, a commitment to your wellbeing, a foundation of your goddess essence. Trust in the process, commit to your journey and watch as your routine becomes a source of strength, joy and transformation.

Now that you're ready to design a routine aligned with your highest self, it's time for the next level: a Menopause Ikigai and Dopamine Menu to infuse your journey with pleasure, joy and divine nourishment. Stay tuned - your goddess glow is about to shine even brighter!

Chapter 10

EMBRACE YOUR GLOW WITH YOUR MENOPAUSE IKIGAI AND DOPAMINE MENU

If you're in the thick of menopause – navigating sleepless nights, sudden emotional waves, or the unsettling sense that your body and mind are shifting in unfamiliar ways – it's completely natural to feel overwhelmed. A woman in her power doesn't ignore these changes. Instead, she acknowledges them, honours them and learns to move through them with wisdom and grace.

Brain fog may cast shadows over your confidence. Your energy might feel like it's disappeared and those glowing moments of joy may seem just out of reach. This season can feel disorienting, but it's also a time of profound transformation. One that invites you to evolve into your most authentic, radiant self.

Two transformational tools will guide you through this divine shift:

The Menopause Ikigai and Dopamine Menu

The **Dopamine Menu** is an intentional, heart-led approach to sparking happiness, motivation and fulfilment in daily life. It's about choosing pleasure, vitality and self-love as your birthright.

Ikigai, the Japanese philosophy of finding your "reason for being" aligns beautifully with the goddess mindset. It encourages you to step into your passion, discover your deeper purpose and create meaning in every stage of life, *especially* in this one.

Together, these sacred practices transform how you experience menopause, helping you feel more grounded, energised and deeply connected to what truly matters.

Your Dopamine Menu for Menopause

Unlike a traditional menu, a dopamine menu isn't just about food. It is a curation of everything that elevates your energy, soothes your soul and reawakens your zest for life. Think of it as your personal empowerment toolkit, blending nourishing nutrition, joyful movement, soul-deep self-care and intentional rituals that ignite your inner fire.

By weaving your Dopamine Menu into the routine we've already explored, you're not just easing menopausal symptoms, you're reclaiming your divine essence, stepping into your radiance and designing a life that uplifts, empowers and energises you every single day.

Let's dive into crafting your personal Menopause Dopamine Menu. Because joy isn't just possible, it's your *divine right.*

What is Dopamine and Why Does It Matter in Menopause?

Dopamine is often referred to as the "feel-good" neurotransmitter because it's deeply connected to pleasure, reward and motivation. It's the surge of satisfaction you feel when you accomplish something, enjoy a delicious meal, or laugh with a loved one.

But during menopause, hormonal shifts can wreak havoc on dopamine levels. With lower oestrogen, disrupted sleep and heightened stress, you may feel drained, unmotivated or simply disconnected from your vibrant self. However, the goddess within you is still very much alive.

By integrating intentional choices into your daily routine, whether through food, physical activity or small acts of self-care, you can boost dopamine production and regain a sense of balance and vitality. The beauty of a Dopamine Menu is its adaptability; it's entirely yours to design.

Creating Your Dopamine Menu

Think of your Dopamine Menu like dining at your favourite restaurant, where every choice is tailored to your tastes. This menu includes quick bites of happiness, deeply satisfying activities, and even indulgent treats. It's flexible and uniquely yours, fitting seamlessly into your routine while adding layers of positivity and pleasure.

Starters: Small Acts, Big Smiles

Picture this: Golden sunlight peeks through your curtains, and instead of diving straight into the day's demands, you put on your favourite song. For the next ten minutes, your kitchen becomes a dance floor, your movements unrestrained and joyful. Dancing isn't just a way to wake your body; it's a chance to wake your spirit, a small act that starts your day with laughter and energy.

Imagine pausing for a moment to sit with your pet. The warmth of their body against yours, their soft fur beneath your fingers. It's a moment of unconditional love that requires nothing but presence.

Or consider the comfort of holding a warm cup of tea, its steam curling upward as you savour each sip, grounding yourself in its simplicity. This is a brief opportunity to centre yourself, to breathe in serenity and exhale anything that no longer serves you.

Perhaps you step outside for a brief moment, barefoot on the grass, connecting with the earth beneath you. Or you take a deep breath and let the crisp morning air fill your lungs, the cold air a reminder that you're here, alive and ready to embrace the day. This grounding practice is a goddess ritual, reminding you of your deep connection to nature's abundant energy. These starters don't demand much of your time, but their impact ripples outward, setting the tone for everything that follows.

Mains: Nourishment for the Soul

Now imagine dedicating time to something more substantial, something that fills you up in ways that linger long after the moment has passed. Perhaps it's an afternoon spent baking a loaf of bread, golden and fragrant, emerging from the oven as a tangible symbol of your effort and care. The kneading of dough becomes almost meditative, each fold and press grounding you in the present.

Khushi finds baking therapeutic. She carves out a couple of hours on a Sunday and relaxes while making the most wonderful focaccia bread – it's drool-worthy, a labour of love, and a moment of delicious, feminine indulgence.

Or picture a walk through a forest or along a quiet path. With each step, the world slows down. You notice the crunch of leaves beneath your feet, the way sunlight filters through branches and the soft melody of birdsong. These walks are more than exercise; they're a chance to reconnect with nature and yourself.

Anjali thrives in nature. Whether she's walking or hiking, moving through the landscape becomes a ritual in itself. She lets her thoughts flow and her heart breathe, embodying the wild feminine energy that finds strength in both motion and stillness.

You might sink into a novel that sweeps you away to another world, the words painting vivid scenes in your mind. Time seems to stop as you lose yourself in the story, emerging later with a sense of renewal and inspiration. Alternatively, it could be an hour of yoga, where the flow of movement and breath quietens your mind and strengthens your body, leaving you feeling both centred and revitalised.

These mains take a bit more time, but their rewards are profound. They ground you, remind you of your strength and create a reservoir of calm and joy to draw from on busier days.

Sides: Elevating Everyday Life

The beauty of sides lies in their simplicity. They don't require you to carve out extra time; instead, they elevate the time you already spend. Picture folding laundry with your favourite podcast playing in the background. The words entertain and inspire you, turning a chore into a moment of enrichment and wisdom.

Or imagine lighting a candle as you sit down to write your to-do list. The flicker of the flame and the delicate scent create a sacred sanctuary amidst the day's busyness. Even washing the dishes can become an act of meditative mindfulness when paired with warm, soapy water and the sound of your favourite playlist in the background.

You might slip into a silken dressing gown as you prepare your morning coffee, turning an ordinary task into a ritual of self-honour. Or take five minutes to water your houseplants, watching the leaves glisten as they soak up the droplets; a gentle reminder of the beauty of nurturing.

Hindae begins her day in reverence, tending to her curry leaf plants with devotion. She checks in with them, offers water, and then flows seamlessly into her morning yoga ritual, aligning body and spirit.

These small gestures transform the mundane into moments of intentional magic, reminding you that joy can be found in even the simplest acts.

Desserts: Savouring Life's Sweetness

Desserts are about indulgence, pleasure and divine delight – those small luxuries that exist simply to be enjoyed. Picture yourself at the end of a long day, slipping into a warm, fragrant bath surrounded by candlelight. As the water embraces you, the weight of the day melts away like honey, leaving only tranquillity and bliss.

Or imagine the soft caress of a plush robe as you move through a skincare ritual steeped in self-devotion. Each step, from the silken glide of facial oil to the gentle sculpting of your face with a gua sha tool, becomes an act of reverence for your body, mind and soul. This is my most cherished self-love ritual, a chance to connect to myself daily.

Perhaps you cocoon yourself in a cosy blanket, allowing space for an episode (or three) of your favourite series – Sasha's divine way to unwind after a long day on her feet.

Desserts are the sweet punctuation marks in your day, moments where you indulge in pleasure simply because it feels good. They're about celebrating yourself and allowing space for joy without guilt.

Specials: Rare but Radiant Moments

Specials are the grand, glittering highlights, the moments that stand out in memory and remind you of life's abundance. Picture a spontaneous weekend trip to the seaside. The salty breeze tousles your hair as the waves crash rhythmically on the shore. You feel the sun on your face, the sand beneath your feet and a sense of freedom that only comes when you step away from your routine.

Or imagine booking a massage at a luxurious spa, where the tension in your body melts away under skilled hands. The tranquillity of the space, the soothing music and the indulgence of being cared for all leave you feeling renewed.

Alex and Dani love spas. There's nothing more luxurious than being pampered after a busy work period. To them, this is a ritual, a moment of pure restoration where they honour their bodies through self-care.

Specials could also be an evening at a fine restaurant, the kind where every bite is a revelation and the atmosphere feels electric with possibility. Or perhaps it's a day spent exploring a new city, each corner revealing something unexpected and beautiful.

These moments don't happen often, but their rarity makes them all the more precious.

They're a reminder of the extraordinary in life and a celebration of the journey you're on.

By crafting and embracing your own Dopamine Menu, you create a life that feels rich, joyful and balanced. These moments, whether small or grand, are all threads in the tapestry of your wellbeing, weaving together a picture of a life well-lived. It's not about perfection; it's about presence, intention and the simple, profound act of choosing joy.

Ikigai: Finding Your Reason for Being

Ikigai (pronounced ee-kee-guy) is a Japanese concept that means "your reason for being". It's about discovering the intersection of what you love, what you're good at, what the world needs and what fulfils you. During menopause, a phase when identity and purpose often feel unsettled, Ikigai can be a transformative mindset tool to help you feel grounded, inspired and empowered.

On Okinawa Island, Japan, people are celebrated for their exceptional longevity and happiness. The World Health Organisation (WHO) notes that Okinawa boasts the highest life expectancy in the world. Their secret? Ikigai: the art of living with soul-aligned purpose.

If like me, you find that the life path you're on no longer resonates - that's perfectly okay. For me, I've had to admit that my calling may never have been the legal profession. A quote that shifted my perspective on my journey and Ikigai is this:

"If you get on the wrong train, get off at the nearest station. The longer you wait, the more expensive the return trip will be."

Read it again. Slowly.

Of course, this isn't just about trains; it's about life.

You're never stuck. You can choose again, pivot and begin anew at any moment. A woman aligned with her inner truth knows she has the power to reinvent herself at any stage. Once you reconnect with that quiet, divine strength within you, everything around you shifts, almost like magic.

When you're living in alignment with your Ikigai, life doesn't have to feel forced. It flows – easily, intuitively, joyfully.

If you're at a crossroads, questioning the trajectory of your life – especially during menopause – let's use Ikigai to reconnect with who you are now.

Why Menopause Is the Perfect Time to Explore Ikigai

Ikigai is powerful because it's like a secret life hack that helps sustain the body, mind and soul. Studies suggest that losing a sense of purpose can impact health, potentially shortening life expectancy, regardless of other healthy habits. Conversely, having a purpose can reduce inflammation and slow cellular ageing.

Menopause isn't just a biological transition; it's also an emotional and spiritual metamorphosis. Instead of seeing menopause as a loss, Ikigai reframes it as an opportunity to focus on what's meaningful.

How Ikigai Shifts Your Mindset During Menopause

Here's how embracing Ikigai can transform how you see this phase of life:

Rediscovering Your Joy

Menopause can sometimes feel like a loss of control, but Ikigai offers a chance to reclaim what truly brings you joy. What are the passions or hobbies that make you feel alive and magnetic? Maybe it's art, writing, gardening or simply spending time in nature. Maybe it's something you haven't done in years but always loved. By focusing on what sets your soul ablaze, Ikigai reminds you that joy is still within reach; you only have to make space for it in your life.

Reframing Your Purpose

It's common during menopause to question your place in the world, especially if your children are grown or your career is shifting. You might ask yourself, *Who am I beyond these past roles? What do I do now?* Ikigai encourages you to see this as a time to awaken a new purpose, not lose one. Instead of focusing on what's behind you, it invites you to look ahead and explore how your unique skills, experiences and passions can continue to bring value to yourself and others.

Creating Emotional Resilience

Menopause often brings emotional turbulence – mood swings, anxiety, or a sense of overwhelm. Ikigai acts as a guiding star, grounding you in what gives your life depth and meaning. It's not about ignoring the challenges but about navigating them with the poise of a goddess.

Strengthening Connections

If menopause feels isolating, Ikigai offers another layer of support by reminding you of the power of connection. What relationships or communities bring you joy? Maybe it's deepening bonds with loved ones, joining a group with shared interests or mentoring someone who could use your wisdom. Building these connections reinforces your sense of purpose and belonging, helping you feel valued and supported.

Caring for Yourself, Inside and Out

Self-care becomes vital during menopause, but it can feel like just another task on your to-do list. Ikigai reframes it as a way to support your purpose. When you take care of your body through movement, nourishment and rest, you're not just managing symptoms, you're creating the energy and balance you need to pursue the things that matter most to you.

What Does Ikigai Look Like for You?

Your Ikigai doesn't have to be grand or world-changing. It just has to feel right for you. Maybe it's creating art, starting a garden, writing your story or mentoring someone who could use your wisdom. Maybe it's taking this time to travel, volunteer or simply slow down and savour life.

Ikigai is about leaning into what brings you fulfilment and joy. It reminds you that menopause isn't the end of your story but rather a new chapter.

So, grab a notebook and take a moment to reflect on these questions:

> What truly matters to me?
> What brings me joy?
> What do I want my life to look like moving forward?

Menopause is a chance to rewrite the narrative. With Ikigai as your guide, you can embrace this phase with purpose, clarity and a sense of empowerment.

A New Beginning

Menopause brings both uncertainty and opportunity. It's a moment to reconnect with yourself, rediscover passions and move into the next chapter with intention.

The next time you're awake in the middle of the night, overwhelmed by change, shift your thoughts like a celestial goddess. Ask yourself, *What brings me joy? How can I lean into that?* That's the beginning of your Ikigai awakening – transforming menopause into a time not just to endure, but to flourish magnificently.

Over the past few years, I have been blessed to meet extraordinary women who have left behind corporate careers to carve out soul-aligned paths. Each finds fulfilment in ways that centre around empowerment, healing and service.

Take Maisha, for example. With a degree in financial planning, she built a career in the financial sector, yet her true calling whispered from beyond the spreadsheets. Answering that call, she embarked on a profound spiritual journey, dedicating herself to ThetaHealing® for over a decade. Her work has not only transformed countless lives but has also deeply shifted my own.

There's Sanaiyah, who left behind an incredible job promotion when she was working as a buyer for a fashion powerhouse to pursue her Ikigai calling towards ThetaHealing® and coaching. Her passion lies in writing and championing self-love to teach clients that they have the power to improve all the relationships around them.

Meet Shalini – a woman of many passions. She transformed her love for wellness into Wholesome Bites, a range of nourishing snacks made with high-quality organic ingredients. But her creativity doesn't stop there. Shalini is also a certified Laughter Yoga facilitator, bringing lightness and laughter into people's lives. Her sessions not only uplift the spirit, but also help reduce stress, boost immunity, and support emotional wellbeing.

Then there's Darpan, who stepped away from the corporate world to champion menopausal women through strength training and holistic nourishment. Her passion lies in guiding women to rediscover their power and feel strong, radiant and sovereign in their own skin.

All of these extraordinary women radiate magnetic, empowering energy, proving that it is never too late to rewrite your destiny.

The lesson? You are not bound to a single path. You can embark on a new journey at any time, at any age. Your next chapter is entirely yours to create.

Bringing Ikigai and a Dopamine Menu Together

The true magic happens when Ikigai and a Dopamine Menu work hand in hand. Ikigai gives your life direction and a clear sense of what sets your soul alight. Meanwhile, your Dopamine Menu keeps you energised, motivated and emotionally resilient as you follow that path.

For example, if your Ikigai involves expressing yourself creatively, you might use your Dopamine Menu to break that goal into smaller, dopamine-rich steps. Spend ten minutes journaling, trying a new art technique or celebrating a completed project with a walk in nature. The small moments of joy from your dopamine menu provide fuel for the bigger, more meaningful pursuits in your life.

When challenges arise, as they inevitably do, the combination of these two tools helps you navigate them with grace. If a sleepless night leaves you feeling irritable or foggy, lean on your dopamine menu. Take a walk, sip tea in the sunlight or listen to an uplifting podcast. These small acts remind you that joy is still within reach, even on the hardest days.

At the same time, your Ikigai keeps you tethered to your purpose. It helps you remember that menopause isn't just a time of loss – it's a chance to explore new passions, deepen your relationships and reconnect with yourself in exciting and meaningful ways.

An Example of Transformation

Imagine waking up after a restless night, your energy low and your mood fragile. Instead of letting the day spiral, you decide to reach for your Dopamine Menu. You start with a gentle stretch, breathing deeply as sunlight streams through the window. Then, you put on an upbeat song and let yourself dance for a few minutes, shaking off the heaviness.

Later in the day, you reflect on your Ikigai and remember how much you've always loved storytelling. You spend twenty minutes journaling, letting your thoughts flow freely. It's not about perfection or productivity; it's about reconnecting with something that brings you joy. By the end of the day, even if your symptoms haven't disappeared, you feel lighter, more purposeful and more in tune with yourself.

Weaving the Dopamine Menu and Ikigai into Your Daily Life

With your Dopamine Menu crafted and your Ikigai discovered, it's time to incorporate these tools into your everyday routine. Together, they form a powerful foundation for creating a productive and joy-filled life, helping you thrive through this transformative phase.

Start by mapping out your week with intention, blending structure with moments of joy. Use your 12-week calendar to schedule activities from your Dopamine Menu. Think of it as planning a menu for your soul: begin your day with a starter like a morning walk to set a positive tone, dedicate evenings to mains such as yoga, baking, or creative pursuits, and sprinkle in sides – simple, nourishing moments like listening to music or savouring a cup of tea.

Tracking your progress can deepen the impact of these practices. Pair your Dopamine Menu and Ikigai with your Menopause Symptoms Tracker, noting which activities you engage in each day and how they make you feel. Over time, patterns will emerge, showing you what best supports your mood, energy and overall wellbeing.

Consistency transforms these practices into rituals that anchor your days. Perhaps every Sunday becomes your "specials" day, a time to indulge in something magical, like a long soak in the bath, crisp fresh linens or a long walk in your favourite park. These rituals create a rhythm to your week, offering moments to look forward to and cherish.

At its heart, the Dopamine Menu is more than just a tool for getting through menopause; it's a way to truly thrive. It allows you to prioritise yourself, embrace the beauty of small joys and find strength in nourishing routines. By aligning these practices with your Ikigai, you're creating a life that feels deeply fulfilling and uniquely yours.

With your Dopamine Menu as a daily source of light and Ikigai as your compass, you're equipped to embrace this new chapter with grace, confidence and a sense of possibility.

So here's to you and the life you're designing. May it be as vibrant, nourishing and empowering as you are.

CONCLUSION
EMBRACING YOUR GLOW

The world has long whispered that ageing is something to fear, that change is something to resist. But here's the truth: Change is inevitable, and your glow is unstoppable. You are not fading; you are ascending. You are stepping into a version of yourself that is wiser, freer and unapologetically authentic. The discomfort, the hot flushes, the emotional tides – these are not signs of loss but signals of renewal. Like a phoenix rising, you are shedding the old to rise into your power.

As you reach the final pages of this book, take a moment to reflect on the incredible goddess journey you've embarked upon. *Glow Through the Change* is more than a guidebook; it's an invitation, a mindset and a promise. Menopause is not an ending but a transformation, a shift into a powerful, luminous new chapter of your life.

Your Power, Your Wisdom

For years, you may have defined yourself by the roles you played – mother, partner, professional, caregiver, friend. Now, the focus turns inward. This is the time to nurture yourself with the same energy and devotion you have so effortlessly given to others. Your wisdom, earned through years of experience, is your most sacred treasure. You have navigated life's storms and still stand strong, resilient and glowing with an inner light that no external force can dim.

Remember that menopause is not a medical condition to be "cured". It is a natural progression, a transition into a phase where your voice grows stronger, your presence bolder, and your intuition sharper. This is the era of self-acceptance, deep and meaningful connections and embracing what brings you joy without guilt or hesitation. You have spent years tending to others. Now, it is time to be the goddess at the centre of your own altar.

The Art of Thriving

To thrive through menopause is not to defy age; it is to define it on your own terms. It is saying "yes" to what fuels your spirit and "no" to what drains your essence. It's about embracing movement, nourishing your body with intention and treating your mind with kindness. It's about surrounding yourself with people who lift you up and walking away from anything that dims your light.

Every choice you make from this point forward is an affirmation of your power. Will you move your body in ways that bring you joy? Will you nourish yourself with food that makes you feel vibrant? Will you set boundaries and honour your needs without apology? The answer lies within you, waiting to be claimed.

Empowering Yourself Through Rituals

You now have all the tools at your fingertips to transform your menopause journey.

You've become your own doctor by using the Menopause Symptoms Tracker to tune into your body and spot the patterns that matter. You've stepped into the role of your own nutritionist, choosing foods that nourish your body, mind and soul with intention. You've taken charge of your wellbeing by bringing gua sha into your daily rhythm – soothing your skin, easing hot flushes, aiding digestion and reducing bloating with care and consistency.

With the 12-week calendar, you've mapped out your goals and anchored them in routine, motivation and mindset. You've prioritised sleep, crafting an evening ritual that restores and recharges you from the inside out.

Every choice you make, every ritual designed and committed to, is a declaration of self-empowerment, allowing you to reclaim control over your menopause journey.

The Power of Gua Sha in Your Menopause Journey

Gua sha is more than just a beauty tool; it's a daily ritual of self-care that allows you to reconnect with your body, honour your emotions and cultivate confidence in your skin. The gentle, rhythmic strokes of gua sha not only help relieve tension and promote circulation but also create a moment of mindfulness, inviting you to slow down and tune into yourself.

As your body changes, this simple practice becomes an act of self-love, a way to nurture your skin and release built-up stress. By incorporating gua sha into your daily routine, you are grounding yourself in self-awareness, embracing your evolving beauty and celebrating the skin you are in.

A Community of Strength

One of the greatest gifts of this stage is the realisation that you are not alone. The sisterhood of women walking this path with you is vast, diverse, and deeply connected. Whether through shared laughter over the unpredictability of hot flushes or heartfelt conversations about the emotions that arise, know that there is strength in solidarity. Seek out and embrace the community that empowers you. Let go of the notion that you must endure this change in silence. Your voice matters, your experiences are valid and your truth deserves to be shared.

If you ever feel uncertain, trust in the strength you have cultivated through this journey. Every step you take toward self-care, self-awareness and self-love reinforces your resilience.

Your Radiant Future

The years ahead are not something to simply endure; they are something to celebrate. Imagine the freedom of embracing yourself fully, of waking up each day without the weight of unrealistic expectations or societal pressures. Picture yourself stepping into your power, speaking your truth and living life with an unshakable confidence. That is the gift of this transition.

You have learned to honour your body, to nourish your soul and to trust your inner wisdom. You have discovered that beauty is not found in youth alone but in the depth of your experiences, the richness of your laughter and the authenticity of your presence. You are glowing – not in spite of menopause, but because of it.

So, take a deep breath and step forward as the goddess you are. Let the world witness your radiance. Stand tall, walk boldly and embrace this magnificent chapter with open arms.

You are strong.
You are wise.
You are luminous.

And most of all, you are ready.

Glow through the change and let the world bask in your divine light.

I would be honoured to walk alongside you for an extra dose of support and confidence as you embrace your journey to your healthiest, glowing self during menopause. Let's connect at www.shanti3.com or on Instagram (@shanti3official) for gua sha rituals, workshops, massages, coaching and holistic wisdom – all designed to help you glow through this beautiful change.

With love and light,
Divya

https://www.instagram.com/shanti3official

https://shanti3.com/pages/book-form

BIBLIOGRAPHY

Books

- Lugo T, Tetrokalashvili M. *Hot flashes*. In: StatPearls [Internet]. Treasure Island (FL): StatPearls Publishing; 19 Dec 2022–. PMID: 30969649.

- Nielsen A. *Gua Sha: A Traditional Technique for Modern Practice*. 2nd ed. United Kingdom: Arya Nielsen; 2012.

Journals

- Aghamohammadi V, Salmani R, Ivanbagha R, Effati Daryani F, Nasiri K. Footbath as a safe, simple, and non-pharmacological method to improve sleep quality of menopausal women. *Res Nurs Health*. Dec 2020;43(6):621–628. doi:10.1002/nur.22082. Epub 28 Oct 2020. PMID: 33112004.

- Curran J. The Yellow Emperor's Classic of Internal Medicine. *BMJ.* 5 Apr 2008;336(7647):777. doi:10.1136/bmj.39527.472303.4E. PMCID: PMC2287209.

- Moradi M, Ghavami V, Niazi A, Seraj Shirvan F, Rasa S. The effect of *Salvia officinalis* on hot flashes in postmenopausal women: a systematic review and meta-analysis. *Int J Community Based Nurs Midwifery.* Jul 2023;11(3):169–178. doi:10.30476/IJCBNM.2023.97639.2198. PMID: 37489230; PMCID: PMC10363264.

- Fang Y, Liu F, Zhang X, et al. Mapping global prevalence of menopausal symptoms among middle-aged women: a systematic review and meta-analysis. *BMC Public Health.* 2024;24:1767.

- Gudise VS, Dasari MP, Kuricheti SSK. Efficacy and safety of *Shatavari* root extract for the management of menopausal symptoms: a double-blind, multicenter, randomized controlled trial. *Cureus.* 8 Apr 2024;16(4):e57879. doi:10.7759/cureus.57879. PMID: 38725785; PMCID: PMC11079574.

- British Menopause. *What is menopause?* [Internet]. Aug 2023 [cited 30 Sep 2024]. Available from: https://thebms.org.uk/wp-content/uploads/2023/08/17-BMS-TfC-What-is-the-menopause-AUGUST2023-A.pdf

- Peacock K, Carlson K, Ketvertis KM. Menopause. In: *StatPearls* [Internet]. Treasure Island (FL): StatPearls Publishing; 21 Dec 2023–. PMID: 29939603.

Websites

- Dewhurst A. *The seven year cycle* [Internet]. [cited 30 Sep 2024]. Available from: https://www.theperiodacupuncturist.co.uk/post/the-seven-year-cycle

- *Breeze through menopause with TCM* [Internet]. [cited 2 Oct 2024]. Available from: https://www.macphersontcm.com/single-post/2019/09/20/breeze-through-menopause-with-tcm

- Kristjansson C. *Traditional Chinese medicine and menopause* [Internet]. [cited 29 Sep 2024]. Available from: https://menoclarity.com/traditional-chinese-medicine-menopause/

- Witham C. *Effective Gua sha techniques for managing hot flashes* [Internet]. [cited 9 Nov 2024]. Available from: https://www.clivewitham.com/single-post/treat-hot-flashes-with-gua-sha

- World Health Organization. *Menopause* [Internet]. [cited 30 Sep 2024]. Available from: https://www.who.int/news-room/fact-sheets/detail/menopause

- The Menopause Charity. *Symptoms list* [Internet]. [cited 9 Oct 2024]. Available from: https://www.themenopausecharity.org/2021/10/21/symptoms-list/

- *The seven-year cycles of women's life according to traditional Chinese medicine* [Internet]. [cited 29 Sep 2024]. Available from: https://acuandherbs.net/the-seven-year-cycles-of-womens-life-according-to-traditional-chinese-medicine/

- Elix Healing. *The 7 year life cycles of women, according to ancient Chinese wisdom* [Internet]. [cited 30 Sep 2024]. Available from: https://elixhealing.com/blogs/the-wisdom/the-7-year-life-cycles-of-women-according-to-tcm?srsltid=AfmBOop4iTMT1EY6aEhJErZi3jhKBzg6zG1NzpNtZw9ZM51qgMv28jto

REFERENCES

Introduction

1. Zhang L, Ruan X, Cui Y, Gu M, Mueck AO: Menopausal symptoms and associated social and environmental factors in midlife Chinese women. Clin Interv Aging. 2020;15:2195–2208. doi: 10.2147/CIA.S278976

Chapter 1

2. Peacock K, Carlson K, Ketvertis KM. Menopause. 21 Dec 2023. In: StatPearls [Internet]. Treasure Island (FL): StatPearls Publishing; Jan 2024–. PMID: 29939603.

3. Fang, Y., Liu, F., Zhang, X. et al. Mapping global prevalence of menopausal symptoms among middle-aged women: a systematic review and meta-analysis. BMC Public Health 24, 1767 (2024).

4. Curran J. The Yellow Emperor's Classic of Internal Medicine. BMJ. 5 Apr 2008;336(7647):777. doi: 10.1136/bmj.39527.472303.4E. PMCID: PMC2287209.

5. 'The Seven-Year Cycles of Women's Life According to Traditional Chinese Medicine' < https://acuandherbs.net/the-seven-year-cycles-of-womens-life-according-to-traditional-chinese-medicine/> accessed 29 September 2024.

6. 'Menopause' < https://www.who.int/news-room/fact-sheets/detail/menopause> accessed 30 September 2024.

7. British Menopause Society, 'What is Menopause?' < https://thebms.org.uk/wp-content/uploads/2023/08/17-BMS-TfC-What-is-the-menopause-AUGUST2023-A.pdf> accessed: 30 September 2024.

8. Fang, Y., Liu, F., Zhang, X. et al. Mapping global prevalence of menopausal symptoms among middle-aged women: a systematic review and meta-analysis. BMC Public Health 24, 1767 (2024).

9. 'Symptoms List' <https://www.themenopausecharity.org/2021/10/21/symptoms-list/> accessed 9 October 2024.

Chapter 2

10. Zouboulis, C. C., Blume-Peytavi, U., Kosmadaki, M., Roó, E., Vexiau-Robert, D., Kerob, D., & Goldstein, S. R. (2022). Skin, hair and beyond: the impact of menopause.

Climacteric, 25(5), 434–442. https://doi.org/10.1080/1369 7137.2022.2050206 pg 435

Chapter 3

11. Moradi M, Ghavami V, Niazi A, Seraj Shirvan F, Rasa S. The Effect of *Salvia* Officinalis on Hot Flashes in Postmenopausal Women: A Systematic Review and Meta-Analysis. Int J Community Based Nurs Midwifery. Jul 2023;11(3):169-178. doi: 10.30476/IJCBNM.2023.97639.2198. Pg 170

12. Gudise VS, Dasari MP, Kuricheti SSK. Efficacy and Safety of Shatavari Root Extract for the Management of Menopausal Symptoms: A Double-Blind, Multicenter, Randomized Controlled Trial. Cureus. 8 Apr 2024;16(4):e57879. doi: 10.7759/cureus.57879. PMID: 38725785; PMCID: PMC11079574.

APPENDIX 1

Your Guide to Menopausal Skincare: Be Confident, Informed and In Control

When it comes to skincare, menopausal skin has its own unique needs: It's drier, more sensitive, and often prone to irritation or hormonal breakouts. With so many products on the market, it's easy to feel overwhelmed or lured in by clever marketing buzzwords like "clean", "natural" or "anti-ageing". But being informed about ingredients can give you the power to make confident, healthy choices for your skin.

This easy list is designed to simplify skincare shopping for menopausal skin. With a focus on natural, nourishing, and effective ingredients, you'll learn what to look for, what to avoid, and how to make decisions that truly serve your skin.

Choose Natural, Skin-Loving Ingredients

Menopausal skin thrives on hydration, protection and repair. Look for these powerhouse ingredients:

- Moisture boosters
  - *Hyaluronic acid* (plant-derived), *glycerine*, and *squalane* to deeply hydrate and combat dryness.

- Plant-based oils
  - *Jojoba oil*: Balances natural oils and nourishes deeply.
  - *Argan oil*: Softens skin and boosts elasticity.
  - *Moringa oil*: Rich in antioxidants, vitamins, and fatty acids for repair.
  - *Sea buckthorn oil*: Brightens and supports skin regeneration.

- Barrier-strengthening actives
  - *Shea butter, ceramides* (plant-based), and *essential fatty acids* repair and protect your skin's natural barrier.

- Antioxidants

  - *Vitamin E, Coenzyme Q10,* and *green tea extract* fight oxidative stress to slow skin ageing.

- Soothing ingredients

  - *Chamomile, rosewater,* and *passionflower* calm redness and irritation.

Why it matters: These ingredients nourish, hydrate, and protect menopausal skin without aggravating sensitivities.

Steer Clear of Common Irritants

Sensitive menopausal skin reacts easily, so avoid these culprits:

- Fragrances

  - Both synthetic and natural fragrances like *linalool* or *limonene* can cause irritation.

- Harsh preservatives

  - Avoid *parabens* and *phenoxyethanol*. Opt for natural alternatives like *rosemary extract* or *vitamin E*.

- Drying alcohols
    - Ingredients like *denatured alcohol* or *ethanol* strip moisture and dehydrate skin.

- Synthetic dyes
    - Artificial colouring has no skin benefit and may trigger reactions.

- Overly processed ingredients
    - Cold-pressed, unrefined oils retain more nutrients and purity.

Why it matters: Irritants worsen dryness and redness, making it essential to choose gentle, skin-friendly options.

Embrace Minimalist, Effective Formulas

Simple skincare is often the most effective. Focus on:

- Short ingredient lists
    - Products with fewer than 10 to 12 high-quality ingredients reduce the risk of irritation.

- Unrefined, cold-pressed oils

    ○ These retain their nutrients for maximum skin benefits.

- Water-free balms or oils

    ○ These are deeply nourishing and often free of unnecessary preservatives.

Why it matters: Thoughtfully formulated products focus on results, not fillers, making them perfect for sensitive skin.

Check Product Formulations and Labels

A little knowledge goes a long way when reading labels:

- Ingredient order

    ○ Ingredients are listed by concentration. If a highlighted ingredient is near the bottom, it's likely included in trace amounts.

- Fragrance-free formulas

    ○ Reduce the risk of irritation by choosing unscented options.

- Low-comedogenic ingredients

  - Choose oils and actives that won't clog pores, especially if hormonal changes cause breakouts.

- Rich, creamy textures

  - Thick creams and balms hydrate deeply and improve elasticity.

- Gentle cleansers

  - Use non-foaming, pH-balanced cleansers that preserve your skin's natural oils.

Why it matters: Understanding formulations ensures you choose effective, irritation-free products.

Test and Monitor Your Skin

Always introduce new products cautiously:

- Patch test first

  - Apply a small amount to your inner arm or jawline and wait 24 hours for any reaction.

- Track your skin's response

    ○ Observe how your skin reacts and adjust as needed to meet its changing needs.

Why it matters: Menopausal skin can be unpredictable. Testing minimises adverse reactions while helping identify what works.

Stay Consistent for Lasting Results

Good skincare takes time and commitment. Remember these tips:

- Stick to a routine

    ○ Natural ingredients may work gradually, but consistency will reward you with healthier, more balanced skin.

- Incorporate relaxation

    ○ Stress affects skin health. Pair your routine with calming rituals like *gua sha* to boost circulation and promote relaxation.

Why it matters: Consistency builds healthier skin and reduces stress, helping you manage hormonal changes more effectively.

APPENDIX 2
50 Essential Ingredients for Menopause-Friendly Meals: Your Ultimate Cheat Sheet

No.	Food	Food Temperature	Flavour	Benefit
1	Apples	Cool	Sweet	Antioxidant-rich; supports digestion and balances meals.
2	Apple Cider Vinegar	Cool	Sour	Aids digestion, supports gut health and helps balance blood sugar levels.
3	Aubergine	Cool	Bitter	High in fibre; supports heart health and helps with oestrogen metabolism.
4	Avocado	Neutral	Sweet	Rich in healthy fats; supports skin health and hormone regulation.

No.	Food	Food Temperature	Flavour	Benefit
5	Barley	Neutral	Sweet	Cooling grain; aids digestion and supports heart health.
6	Berries	Cool	Sweet	High in antioxidants; supports brain health and reduces inflammation.
7	Broccoli	Neutral	Bitter	Supports oestrogen metabolism and detoxification; high in antioxidants.
8	Brussel Sprouts	Neutral	Bitter	High in antioxidants; supports hormonal health and detoxification.
9	Cabbage	Cold	Sweet	High in fibre and antioxidants; supports digestion and reduces inflammation.
10	Carrots	Neutral	Sweet	High in beta-carotene; supports skin health and boosts collagen production.
11	Cauliflower	Neutral	Bitter	Supports detoxification and oestrogen metabolism.

No.	Food	Food Temperature	Flavour	Benefit
12	Celery	Cold	Sweet	Hydrating and cooling; reduces body heat and supports digestion.
13	Chickpeas	Neutral	Sweet	High in fibre and protein; supports digestion and hormone balance.
14	Chilli Peppers	Hot	Pungent	Boosts metabolism and improves circulation.
15	Coriander	Cool	Bitter	Aids detoxification, reduces bloating and supports digestion.
16	Edamame	Cool	Sweet	Protein-rich and cooling; supports hormone balance.
17	Flaxseeds	Neutral	Bitter	Rich in lignans; supports hormone balance and heart health.
18	Garlic	Warm	Pungent	Boosts immunity, supports cardiovascular health and has anti-inflammatory properties.
19	Ginger	Warm	Pungent	Boosts circulation, aids digestion and reduces inflammation.

No.	Food	Food Temperature	Flavour	Benefit
20	Green Beans	Neutral	Sweet	High in fibre and vitamins; supports digestion.
21	Green Tea	Cool	Bitter	Antioxidant-rich; reduces inflammation and helps regulate body temperature.
22	Honey	Warm	Sweet	Natural energy booster; supports immunity.
23	Kefir	Cool	Sour	Probiotic-rich; supports gut health and immunity.
24	Kale	Neutral	Bitter	High in fibre and vitamins; aids digestion and supports hormone balance.
25	Kimchi	Cool	Salty	Fermented; promotes gut health and provides probiotics.
26	Lemons	Cold	Sour	High in Vitamin C; aids digestion and boosts immunity.
27	Lentils	Neutral	Sweet	Rich in protein and fibre; supports heart and gut health.
28	Miso	Neutral	Salty	Fermented; rich in probiotics for gut health and supports digestion.
29	Oats	Neutral	Sweet	High in fibre; supports digestion and provides long-lasting energy.

No.	Food	Food Temperature	Flavour	Benefit
30	Okra	Neutral	Bitter	Rich in fibre and antioxidants; supports gut health, aids digestion and improves skin.
31	Onion	Warm	Pungent	Aids circulation, boosts immunity and adds pungency to meals.
32	Oranges	Cool	Sour	High in Vitamin C; boosts immunity and reduces inflammation.
33	Pak Choi	Cold	Sweet	High in antioxidants; natural coolant and supports digestion.
34	Parsley	Cool	Bitter	Aids in detoxification and supports kidney health.
35	Peas	Neutral	Sweet	High in protein, fibre and phytoestrogens; supports digestion and hormonal balance.
36	Peppers	Warm	Pungent	High in Vitamin C; boosts immunity and promotes healthy skin.
37	Pickles	Cool	Salty	Fermented; promotes gut health and digestion.
38	Prunes	Neutral	Sweet	High in fibre; supports digestion and bone health.
39	Rice	Neutral	Sweet	Provides energy and balances meals with its neutral temperature.

No.	Food	Food Temperature	Flavour	Benefit
40	Seaweed	Cool	Salty	High in iodine; supports thyroid health, metabolism and provides essential minerals.
41	Sesame Seeds	Warm	Bitter	High in healthy fats; supports hormone regulation.
42	Soy	Neutral	Sweet	Phytoestrogen; alleviates hot flushes, supports bone health and balances hormones.
43	Spinach	Neutral	Bitter	Rich in iron and magnesium; supports energy levels and bone health.
44	Sweet Potatoes	Neutral	Sweet	Rich in fibre and beta-carotene; supports digestion and skin health.
45	Tofu	Neutral	Sweet	High in protein and phytoestrogens; balances hormones.
46	Tomatoes	Cool	Sour	Lycopene-rich; reduces inflammation and supports heart health.
47	Turmeric	Warm	Bitter	Anti-inflammatory; supports joint health and reduces oxidative stress.
48	Walnuts	Neutral	Bitter	Rich in omega-3 fats; supports brain and hormonal health.

No.	Food	Food Temperature	Flavour	Benefit
49	Watermelon	Cold	Sweet	Hydrating; natural coolant for hot flushes and promotes kidney health.
50	Wheat	Neutral	Sweet	High in fibre; supports gut health and energy levels.

Printed in Dunstable, United Kingdom